Update in Sexually Transmitted Infections

Editor

JEANNE M. MARRAZZO

INFECTIOUS DISEASE CLINICS OF NORTH AMERICA

www.id.theclinics.com

Consulting Editor
HELEN W. BOUCHER

December 2013 • Volume 27 • Number 4

ELSEVIER

1600 John F. Kennedy Boulevard • Suite 1800 • Philadelphia, Pennsylvania, 19103-2899.
http://www.theclinics.com

INFECTIOUS DISEASE CLINICS OF NORTH AMERICA Volume 27, Number 4
December 2013 ISSN 0891–5520, ISBN-13: 978-0-323-26102-9

Editor: Jessica McCool
Developmental Editor: Donald Mumford

Infectious Disease Clinics of North America (ISSN 0891–5520) is published in March, June, September, and December by Elsevier Inc., 360 Park Avenue South, New York, NY 10010-1710. Periodicals postage paid at New York, NY and additional mailing offices. Subscription prices are $295.00 per year for US individuals, $510.00 per year for US institutions, $145.00 per year for US students, $350.00 per year for Canadian individuals, $638.00 per year for Canadian institutions, $420.00 per year for international individuals, $638.00 per year for international institutions, and $200.00 per year for Canadian and international students. To receive student rate, orders must be accompanied by name of affiliated institution, date of term, and the *signature* of program/residency coordinator on institution letterhead. Orders will be billed at individual rate until proof of status is received. Foreign air speed delivery is included in all *Clinics* subscription prices. All prices are subject to change without notice. **POSTMASTER**: Send address changes to *Infectious Disease Clinics of North America,* Elsevier Health Sciences Division, Subcription Customer Service, 3251 Riverport Lane, Maryland Heights, MO 63043. **Customer Service: 1-800-654-2452 (US). From outside of the US and Canada, call 1-314-447-8871. Fax: 1-314-447-8029. E-mail: JournalsCustomerService-usa@elsevier.com (print support) or JournalsOnlineSupport-usa@elsevier.com (online support).**

Infectious Disease Clinics of North America is also published in Spanish by Editorial Inter-Médica, Junin 917, 1er A 1113, Buenos Aires, Argentina.

Reprints. For copies of 100 or more, of articles in this publication, please contact the Commercial Reprints Department, Elsevier Inc., 360 Park Avenue South, New York, New York 10010-1710. Tel. 212-633-3874, Fax: 212-633-3820, E-mail: reprints@elsevier.com.

Infectious Disease Clinics of North America is covered in *MEDLINE/PubMed (Index Medicus), Current Contents/ Clinical Medicine, Science Citation Alert, SCISEARCH,* and *Research Alert.*

Printed and bound by CPI Group (UK) Ltd, Croydon, CR0 4YY

Contributors

CONSULTING EDITOR

HELEN W. BOUCHER, MD, FIDSA, FACP
Director, Infectious Diseases Fellowship Program; Associate Professor of Medicine, Division of Geographic Medicine and Infectious Diseases, Tufts Medical Center, Boston, Massachusetts

EDITOR

JEANNE M. MARRAZZO, MD, MPH
Professor, Division of Allergy and Infectious Diseases, Medical Director, Seattle STD/HIV Prevention Training Center (PTC), Harborview Medical Center, University of Washington, Seattle, Washington

AUTHORS

LINDLEY A. BARBEE, MD, MPH
Senior Fellow, Department of Medicine, Division of Allergy and Infectious Diseases, University of Washington; Assistant Medical Director of STD Program, HIV/STD Program, Public Health – Seattle and King County, Seattle, Washington

STEPHANIE E. COHEN, MD, MPH
Population Health Division, Medical Director, San Francisco City Clinic, San Francisco Department of Public Health; Assistant Clinical Professor, Division of Infectious Diseases, University of California, San Francisco, San Francisco, California

JULIA C. DOMBROWSKI, MD, MPH
Assistant Professor, Department of Medicine, Division of Allergy and Infectious Diseases, University of Washington; Deputy Director for Clinical Services, HIV/STD Program, Public Health – Seattle and King County, Seattle, Washington

EILEEN F. DUNNE, MD, MPH
Medical Epidemiologist, Division of STD Prevention, Centers for Disease Control and Prevention, Atlanta, Georgia

JOSEPH ENGELMAN, MD
Population Health Division, Physician Specialist, San Francisco City Clinic, San Francisco Department of Public Health; Professor of Medicine, Department of Epidemiology and Biostatistics, University of California, San Francisco, San Francisco, California

LINDA GORGOS, MD, MSc
Special Immunology Associates, El Rio Health Center, Tucson, Arizona

JEFFREY D. KLAUSNER, MD, MPH
Professor of Medicine and Public Health, David Geffen School of Medicine, Jonathan and Karin Fielding School of Public Health, University of California, Los Angeles, Los Angeles, California

LISA E. MANHART, PhD
Associate Professor, Departments of Epidemiology and Global Health, University of Washington, Seattle, Washington

JEANNE M. MARRAZZO, MD, MPH
Professor, Division of Allergy and Infectious Diseases, Medical Director, Seattle STD/HIV Prevention Training Center (PTC), Harborview Medical Center, University of Washington, Seattle, Washington

ELISSA MEITES, MD, MPH
Division of STD Prevention, National Center for HIV, Viral Hepatitis, STD, and TB Prevention, Centers for Disease Control and Prevention, Atlanta, Georgia

CAROLINE MITCHELL, MD, MPH
Assistant Professor, Department of Obstetrics and Gynecology, University of Washington, Seattle, Washington

INA U. PARK, MD, MS
Assistant Professor, Department of Family and Community Medicine, University of California, San Francisco School of Medicine, San Francisco; Medical Director, California STD/HIV Prevention Training Center, Oakland, California

SUSAN PHILIP, MD, MPH
Director, Disease Control and Prevention, Population Health Division, San Francisco Department of Public Health; Assistant Clinical Professor, Division of Infectious Diseases, University of California, San Francisco, San Francisco, California

MALAVIKA PRABHU, MD
Resident, Department of Obstetrics and Gynecology, University of Washington, Seattle, Washington

DEVIKA SINGH, MD, MPH
Department of Global Health, Faculty, Seattle STD/HIV Prevention Training Center (PTC), University of Washington, Seattle, Washington

Contents

Preface: Sexually Transmitted Infections   ix

Jeanne M. Marrazzo

Syphilis in the Modern Era: An Update for Physicians   705

Stephanie E. Cohen, Jeffrey D. Klausner, Joseph Engelman, and Susan Philip

> Syphilis is a complex, systemic disease caused by the spirochete *Treponema pallidum*. Syphilis is most commonly transmitted sexually or congenitally and can involve nearly every organ system. Its clinical progression involves several well-characterized stages: an incubation period, a primary stage, a secondary stage, a latent stage, and a late or tertiary stage. Syphilis during pregnancy is a leading cause of perinatal mortality in sub-Saharan Africa and can cause spontaneous abortion, stillbirth, prematurity, low birth weight, or congenital syphilis. Penicillin is highly effective against syphilis and remains the treatment of choice. This article reviews the epidemiology, clinical features, diagnostic approach, treatment, and prevention of syphilis.

Control of *Neisseria gonorrhoeae* in the Era of Evolving Antimicrobial Resistance   723

Lindley A. Barbee and Julia C. Dombrowski

> *Neisseria gonorrhoeae* has developed resistance to all previous first-line antimicrobial therapies over the past 75 years. Today the cephalosporins, the last available antibiotic class that is sufficiently effective, are also threatened by evolving resistance. Screening for asymptomatic gonorrhea in women and men who have sex with men, treating with a dual antibiotic regimen, ensuring effective partner therapy, and remaining vigilant for treatment failures constitute critical activities for clinicians in responding to evolving antimicrobial resistance. This article reviews the epidemiology, history of antimicrobial resistance, current screening and treatment guidelines, and future treatment options for gonorrhea.

Screening and Management of Genital Chlamydial Infections   739

Devika Singh and Jeanne M. Marrazzo

> Chlamydial genital infection is common and asymptomatic in most cases. National screening efforts developed to educate practitioners, expand screening, and link testing to local health laboratories are not meeting the needs of populations at great risk of disease, including young racial/ethnic minority women and sexual minorities. The development and availability of newer diagnostics will likely make chlamydia testing more efficient and widely available for patients and providers. Practitioners are reminded to have a low threshold to offer testing and presumptive treatment to patients that are deemed at high risk of disease, particularly those who are challenging to engage in care.

Trichomoniasis: The "Neglected" Sexually Transmitted Disease   755

Elissa Meites

Trichomonas vaginalis is the most prevalent nonviral sexually transmitted infection, affecting an estimated 3.7 million people in the United States. Although trichomoniasis is common, it has been considered a "neglected" sexually transmitted disease, due to limited knowledge of its sequelae and associated costs. This article reviews current epidemiology, pathophysiology, diagnostic methods, clinical management recommendations and special considerations, research on associated conditions and costs, prevention strategies, and controversies regarding trichomoniasis.

HPV and HPV-Associated Diseases   765

Eileen F. Dunne and Ina U. Park

Human papillomavirus (HPV) is the most common sexually transmitted infection. HPV is associated with a significant burden of disease and cancer, including anogenital warts and recurrent respiratory papillomatosis, and anogenital and oropharyngeal cancers. Effective prevention is available, including primary prevention of cancers and anogenital warts through HPV vaccination, and secondary prevention of cervical cancer through screening and treatment of precancer. This article focuses on HPV infection and the clinical consequences of infection, with attention to cervical and anogenital squamous intraepithelial neoplasia and anogenital warts.

Mycoplasma genitalium: An Emergent Sexually Transmitted Disease?   779

Lisa E. Manhart

This article summarizes the epidemiologic evidence linking Mycoplasma genitalium to sexually transmitted disease syndromes, including male urethritis, and female cervicitis, pelvic inflammatory disease, infertility, and adverse birth outcomes. It discusses the relationship of this bacterium to human immunodeficiency virus infection and reviews the available literature on the efficacy of standard antimicrobial therapies against M genitalium.

Pelvic Inflammatory Disease: Current Concepts in Pathogenesis, Diagnosis and Treatment   793

Caroline Mitchell and Malavika Prabhu

Pelvic inflammatory disease (PID) is characterized by infection and inflammation of the upper genital tract in women and can cause significant reproductive health sequelae for women. Although a definitive diagnosis of PID is made by laparoscopic visualization of inflamed, purulent fallopian tubes, PID is generally a clinical diagnosis and thus represents a diagnostic challenge. Therefore, diagnosis and treatment algorithms advise a high index of suspicion for PID in any woman of reproductive age with pelvic or abdominal pain. Antibiotic therapy should be started early, and given for an adequate period of time to reduce the risk of complications. Coverage for anaerobic organisms should be considered in most cases.

Sexual Transmission of Viral Hepatitis   **811**

Linda Gorgos

Identification and vaccination of adults at risk for hepatitis B virus acquisition through sexual contact is a key strategy to reduce new hepatitis B virus infections among at-risk adults. Hepatitis C has emerged as a sexually transmitted infection among men with male sex partners (MSM). Several biological and behavioral factors have been linked to hepatitis C virus transmission among MSM, including human immunodeficiency virus coinfection; participation in sexual practices that result in mucosal damage or result in exposure to blood; presence of sexually transmitted diseases (STIs), particularly ulcerative STIs; multiple/casual sex partners; and unprotected anal intercourse.

Index   **837**

INFECTIOUS DISEASE CLINICS OF NORTH AMERICA

FORTHCOMING ISSUES

March 2014
Urinary Tract Infections
Kalpana Gupta, *Editor*

June 2014
Antimicrobial Stewardship
Pranita Tamma, Arjun Srinivasan,
and Sara Cosgrove, *Editors*

September 2014
Updates in HIV/AIDS, Part I
Michael S. Saag, and
Henry Masur, *Editors*

RECENT ISSUES

September 2013
**Foodborne Illness: Latest Threats
and Emerging Issues**
David Acheson,
Jennifer McEntire, and
Cheleste M. Thorpe, *Editors*

June 2013
**Infectious Disease Challenges in Solid
Organ Transplant Recipients**
Joseph G. Timpone Jr and
Princy N. Kumar, *Editors*

March 2013
**Community-Acquired Pneumonia:
Controversies and Questions**
Thomas M. File Jr, *Editor*

RELATED INTEREST

Medical Clinics of North America, July 2013 (Vol. 97, Issue 4)
Infectious Disease Threats
Douglas S. Paauw, *Editor*
Available at: http://www.medical.theclinics.com/

**DOWNLOAD
Free App!**

Review Articles
THE CLINICS

NOW AVAILABLE FOR YOUR iPhone and iPad

Preface

Sexually Transmitted Infections

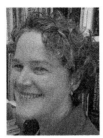

Jeanne M. Marrazzo, MD, MPH
Editor

The need for effective prevention and management of sexually transmitted diseases (STI) continues to be as compelling as it was in the pre-AIDS era. In the United States, most new HIV infections continue to occur in men who have sex with men (MSM), a population that also now has the highest incidence of syphilis—an infection many clinicians had experience with primarily in the pre-AIDS era, and one completely new to many young clinicians. This protean disease continues to present diagnostic and management challenges to those who care for patients at risk, particularly when coinfection with HIV is involved. Rates of other reportable STI either have not declined or have actually increased in the last decade. In 2011, more than 1.4 million cases of *Clamydia trachomatis* were reported to the Centers for Disease Control and Prevention (CDC). Despite this, interventions to detect this common infection in populations most at risk are infrequently performed. Rates of routine annual screening for genital chlamydial infections in young women, especially adolescents, remain suboptimal, and many women at low risk (primarily those over age 30 years without other indications) are tested unnecessarily. Moreover, recommendations to routinely retest infected persons 4 to 6 months after treatment (a practice termed repeat testing, which is distinct from test-of-cure) are not frequently adhered to—despite the fact that this approach detects repeat infection in approximately 15% to 40% of those tested.

The relentless evolution of antimicrobial resistance in *Neisseria gonorrhoeae* continues to present a major challenge. Fluoroquinolones are no longer effective due to widespread resistance, a trend especially notable in MSM. We are now effectively left with only a single class of antibiotics—the cephalosporins—that reliably treat this infection. Concern for nascent development of resistance to this class is looming. Finally, sexual transmission of hepatitis C has been increasingly recognized in MSM who report sexual practices involving exposure to blood or even minimal trauma to the rectal mucosa.

Infect Dis Clin N Am 27 (2013) ix–x
http://dx.doi.org/10.1016/j.idc.2013.09.007
0891-5520/13/$ – see front matter © 2013 Elsevier Inc. All rights reserved.
id.theclinics.com

These worrisome trends emphasize the need for physicians to be aware of emerging STI-related challenges, and of the availability of guidelines and tools to help manage their patients. The CDC Sexually Transmitted Disease Treatment Guidelines are available at www.cdc.gov/std/treatment and are an invaluable resource. As reviewed in the following articles, positive developments include the licensure immunization against several common genital human papillomavirus types for women and men. Against the backdrop of providing key epidemiologic trends for each disease, the authors have emphasized that clinical recognition and diagnosis of these infections are not always straightforward. Moreover, therapeutic management of some STI can be complicated by limited diagnostic capability, coinfections, and immune compromise due to HIV infection. In addition to biomedical management of the individual patient who is affected by STI, clinicians must remember that prevention of these infections requires combinations of biomedical, behavioral, and structural interventions.

Jeanne M. Marrazzo, MD, MPH
Division of Allergy & Infectious Diseases
Seattle STD/HIV Prevention Training Center
University of Washington
Box 359932, Harborview Medical Center, 325 9th Avenue
Seattle, WA 98104, USA

E-mail address:
jmm2@uw.edu

SELECTED READINGS

Centers for Disease Control and Prevention. Sexually transmitted disease treatment guidelines. MMWR Recomm Rep 2010;59.
Wandeler G, Gsponer T, Bregenzer A, et al. Hepatitis C virus infections in the Swiss HIV Cohort Study: a rapidly evolving epidemic. Clin Infect Dis 2012;55:1408–16.
Workowski KA, Berman S, Centers for Disease Control and Prevention (CDC). Sexually transmitted diseases treatment guidelines, 2010. MMWR Recomm Rep 2010; 59:1–110.

Syphilis in the Modern Era
An Update for Physicians

Stephanie E. Cohen, MD, MPH[a],*, Jeffrey D. Klausner, MD, MPH[b],
Joseph Engelman, MD[a], Susan Philip, MD, MPH[c]

KEYWORDS

- Sexually transmitted disease • Syphilis • *Treponema pallidum* • Chancre
- Men who have sex with men • Benzathine penicillin G

KEY POINTS

- Syphilis is common among men who have sex with men and is associated with HIV acquisition.
- Syphilis can cause a wide range of systemic manifestations.
- Penicillin G remains the treatment of choice for all stages of syphilis.
- Syphilis partner services and presumptive treatment of contacts based on exposure history is essential to prevent syphilis reinfection and control the spread of disease.

ETIOLOGY AND PATHOGENESIS

Syphilis is caused by infection with the spirochetal bacterium *Treponema* subspecies *pallidum*. *T pallidum* is a highly motile coiled organism with tapering ends and 6 to 14 spirals. Of uniform cylindrical shape, the bacteria measure approximately 6 to 15 μm in length and 0.25 μm in width. *T pallidum* is a slowly metabolizing organism with an average multiplication time of approximately 30 hours. Humans are the only host for the organism.[1] Most cases of syphilis are transmitted by sexual contact (vaginal, anogenital, and orogenital), but it can also be spread congenitally (in utero or less

Disclosures: J. Engelman has nothing to disclose. S.E. Cohen has received research support from the US National Institutes of Health. In the past year, S. Philip has received research support from Roche Diagnostics, SeraCare Inc, Abbott Diagnostics, and Cepheid Inc. J.D. Klausner has received educational and research support from Hologic Gen-Probe Inc, Cepheid Inc, Standard Diagnostics, Inc, and the US National Institutes of Health.
[a] Population Health Division, San Francisco City Clinic, San Francisco Department of Public Health, 356 7th Street, San Francisco, CA 94103, USA; [b] David Geffen School of Medicine, Jonathan and Karin Fielding School of Public Health, University of California Los Angeles, 9911 West Pico Boulevard, Los Angeles, CA 90049, USA; [c] Population Health Division, San Francisco Department of Public Health, 1360 Mission Street, Suite 401, San Francisco, CA 94103, USA
* Corresponding author.
E-mail address: Stephanie.cohen@sfdph.org

Infect Dis Clin N Am 27 (2013) 705–722
http://dx.doi.org/10.1016/j.idc.2013.08.005
0891-5520/13/$ – see front matter © 2013 Elsevier Inc. All rights reserved.

id.theclinics.com

commonly during passage through the birth canal).[2–4] Rare cases of acquisition through blood products have also been reported.[5–7] On skin-to-skin contact the motile spirochetes enter through areas of microtrauma of the skin or mucosa, multiplying locally with resultant systemic dissemination within 24 hours. The phospholipid-rich outer membrane of the spirochete contains few surface-exposed proteins; this may help it evade the host immune system. The primary pathologic lesion, found at all stages of the disease, is an obliterative endarteritis that leads to many of the clinical manifestations of syphilis. Histologic examination of a chancre is characterized by an intense infiltrate of plasma cells, with scattered macrophages and lymphocytes. A granulomatous reaction can also occur.[8]

EPIDEMIOLOGY

Infectious syphilis reached a historic low in the United States in 2000, with only 9756 primary and secondary cases (2.1 per 100,000 persons) compared with approximately 100,000 cases (71 per 100,000 persons) in 1946.[9] In response to declining syphilis incidence, the Centers for Disease Control and Prevention released "The National Plan to Eliminate Syphilis from the United States" in 1999.[10] However, starting in 2001, rates of primary and secondary syphilis have continued to rise, with an epidemic resurgence among men who have sex with men (MSM) (**Fig. 1**).[9,11] In 2011, there were 13,970 primary and secondary syphilis cases in the United States (4.5 per 100,000 persons), and 72% of cases for which there was information about gender of sex partners were among MSM. Reversal in the control of syphilis in disenfranchised, low socioeconomic black heterosexual subpopulations has also been observed in major metropolitan areas in the Southeast of the United States.[9] In San Francisco and many other large urban areas that have experienced increases in the incidence of syphilis among MSM, approximately two-third of cases occur in HIV-infected men; HIV incidence among HIV-uninfected men with syphilis is high.[12–15] Similar trends in syphilis have been reported throughout Europe in cities with large populations of MSM.[16,17]

The syphilis epidemic among MSM has been attributed to individual, network, and population level factors, including (1) a decrease in safer sex practices secondary to HIV prevention fatigue, antiretroviral treatment optimism, and an increase in recreational drug use, especially methamphetamines and erectile dysfunction

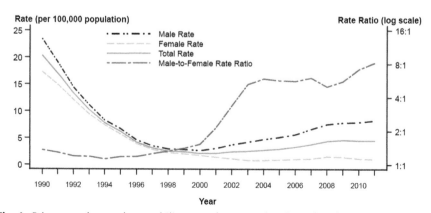

Fig. 1. Primary and secondary syphilis—rates by sex and male-to-female rate ratios, United States, 1990–2011. (*From* Centers for Disease Control and Prevention, December 2012. Available at: http://www.cdc.gov/std/stats11/figures/38.htm. Accessed June 21, 2013.)

medications; (2) harm-reduction strategies like serosorting (selective unprotected sex with partners of the same HIV-serostatus) and oral sex, which may decrease the risk of HIV transmission but can facilitate syphilis transmission; (3) rising use of the Internet as a meeting venue, which has revolutionized sexual networks and facilitated sex partnering, leading to increased number of sex partners, including anonymous partners who cannot be reached for partner services; and (4) decreasing AIDS mortality, which has increased the size of the population at risk for syphilis.[13,18–26] Rising antiretroviral coverage suppresses individual and community HIV viral load and prevents HIV but not syphilis transmission. This may partially explain the divergence between HIV and syphilis rates among MSM that is occurring in some municipalities.[27,28] If other biomedical HIV-prevention strategies, for instance pre-exposure prophylaxis, become more widespread, the divergence between syphilis and HIV epidemiology may further widen.

Syphilis is endemic throughout the developing world. Regional data from the World Health Organization demonstrate that approximately 5% of pregnant women seeking antenatal care services in the Western Pacific, Sub-Saharan Africa, South Asia, and South America have evidence of recent syphilis infection. This results in a substantial burden of adverse pregnancy outcomes, such as miscarriages, stillbirths, and newborns with congenital syphilis infection. An estimated 1.4 million pregnancies are affected annually worldwide. Globally, congenital syphilis is more common than perinatal HIV infection.[29]

The well-documented increase of syphilis in China has intensified global concern about syphilis. An aggressive venereal disease control policy of the Chinese government during the 1950s to 1970s effectively eliminated syphilis, but recent data show a 250- to 1000-fold increase in adult and congenital cases, respectively, in the last decade.[30] This is thought to be caused by several sociopolitical, economic, and cultural factors, including skewed sex ratios in some communities, a large rural-to-urban migrant population, expanding demand for commercial sex, stigma related to same sex behaviors, and low use of sexual health services.[31]

HISTORICAL PERSPECTIVE

Current understanding of the natural course of syphilis infection among untreated individuals is largely based on historical data from the preantibiotic era. The Oslo Study was a large prospective natural history study in which Boeck observed approximately 2000 patients with primary and secondary syphilis admitted to the Oslo Clinic from 1891 to 1910.[32] From 1932 to 1972 in Macon County, Alabama, the US Public Health Service conducted the infamous Tuskegee Syphilis Study to observe untreated syphilis infection among African American men. Treatment was withheld from study participants even after the discovery of penicillin. Lessons learned from the Tuskegee Study have shaped modern standards regarding research ethics and informed consent.[33] In 2008, Susan Reverby, a historian and expert on the Tuskegee Study, discovered that the US Public Health Service exposed several hundred Guatemalans, many of whom were prisoners, sex workers, or patients in a mental institution, to syphilis in an undocumented research project in 1946 to 1948. The horrific ethical violations that transpired led to an official apology from the United States to the Guatemalan government and an investigation by the Presidential Commission on Bioethical issues. Those studies provide important reminders that the quest for answers in biomedical research can blind researchers to moral concerns and the rights of study participants, and underscore the importance of bioethics training, community advisory boards, and institutional review boards.[34,35]

CLINICAL FEATURES
Early Syphilis

Early syphilis, which includes the primary, secondary, and early latent stages of infection, is defined as syphilis of less than 1 year's duration. That designation is based on the observation that infectivity declines after the first year.

Primary syphilis

Primary syphilis presents 1 week to 3 months (median, 21 days) after exposure with a painless lesion, a chancre, at the site of inoculation and nontender regional lymphadenopathy. The lesion starts as a papule and rapidly forms an ulcer that is typically nonexudative with a clean base (**Fig. 2**). Primary lesions are most commonly found on the external genitalia, but can develop on any site of exposure including the perineum, cervix, anus, rectum, lips, oropharynx, and hands (**Figs. 3** and **4**). Multiple chancres can occur and are more common in patients with HIV infection (**Fig. 5**). Without treatment, the chancre usually heals on its own within 1 to 3 weeks.[36] Primary syphilis must be differentiated from other causes of genital ulcer disease including other infectious causes (herpes simplex virus, chancroid, lymphogranuloma venereum, and pyogenic ulcers) and noninfectious causes (trauma, neoplasia, and fixed drug eruptions). Herpetic ulcers, unlike chancres, are usually superficial, vesicular, nonindurated, and painful. Chancroid, caused by *Haemophilus ducreyi*, is rare in the United States and is typically nonindurated, painful, and exudative with a necrotic base.

Secondary syphilis

The timing of onset of the secondary stage of syphilis is highly variable. It typically occurs 2 to 8 weeks after the disappearance of a chancre, but in some cases the primary chancre may still be present. Many patients do not recall a history of a primary lesion. Secondary syphilis typically presents with rash, fever, headache, pharyngitis, and lymphadenopathy, but has a wide range of possible systemic manifestations including hepatitis, glomerulonephritis, periostitis, and early neurologic complications, such as uveitis and meningitis.[36]

The cutaneous manifestations of secondary syphilis are diverse. The classic exanthem of secondary syphilis is a diffuse maculopapular rash that often, but not always, involves the palms and soles (**Fig. 6**) and scrotum (**Fig. 7**). However, the rash can also be papular, annular, or pustular, and can have a fine overlying scale. Other mucocutaneous manifestations include (1) condylomata lata (moist heaped-up broad plaques found in intertriginous areas, such as the perianal area, vulva, and inner thighs; **Fig. 8**); (2) mucous patches (gray, superficial erosions or plaques on the buccal mucosa and tongue, under the prepuce, and on the inner labia; **Fig. 9**); (3) split papules (fissured, nodular lesions at the angle of the lips and in the nasolabial folds; **Fig. 10**); and (4)

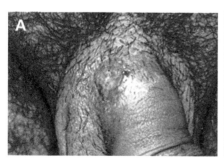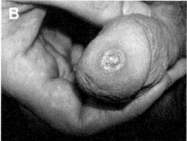

Fig. 2. (*A, B*) Penile chancres.

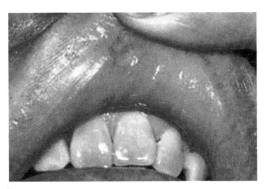

Fig. 3. Chancre on lip.

patchy alopecia (thinning of hair, eyebrows, and beard caused by syphilitic involvement of the hair follicle). The cutaneous lesions of syphilis, particularly the nonkeratinized mucocutaneous lesions (condylomata lata and mucous patches), contain large concentrations of spirochetes and are highly infectious.

Invasion of the central nervous system (CNS) is common during secondary syphilis, and may be asymptomatic or may manifest as an aseptic meningitis, with headache, neck stiffness, and a lymphocytic pleocytosis of cerebrospinal fluid (CSF). The meningeal inflammation is often basilar, leading to unilateral or bilateral cranial nerve abnormalities, particularly of cranial nerves II, III, VI, VII, and VIII.

The diverse manifestations of secondary syphilis earn it the name "the great imitator." Other diseases that should be considered in the differential diagnosis of fever, rash, pharyngitis, and lymphadenopathy include mononucleosis (acute Epstein-Barr virus infection); acute HIV infection; and other viral syndromes. The condylomata lata of secondary syphilis should be distinguished from condylomata acuminata (multiple, small, raised genital warts caused by human papilloma virus). Mucous patches can be mistaken for oral candidiasis. Other infections that cause a rash involving the palms and soles include Rocky Mountain spotted fever; meningococcemia; measles; and certain coxsackievirus infections (hand-foot-and-mouth disease).

Early latent syphilis
Without treatment, the manifestations of secondary syphilis generally resolve within a few weeks. The disease then enters a latent phase, characterized by a lack of clinical

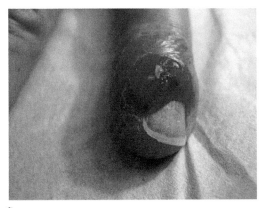

Fig. 4. Chancre on finger.

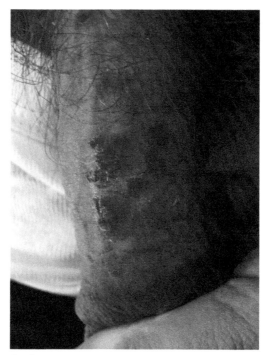

Fig. 5. Multiple penile chancres.

signs of syphilis but positive serologic tests. Observational studies have shown that recrudescent secondary syphilis symptoms can occur in untreated patients up to 5 years after their initial presentation, but generally these relapses occur within the first year. Early latency has therefore been defined as the asymptomatic period during the first year after initial syphilis infection. A patient who is found to have a reactive serologic test for syphilis can be diagnosed as having early latent syphilis if, during the prior year, they had (1) a documented nonreactive serologic test or fourfold or greater increase in titer of a nontreponemal test; (2) unequivocal symptoms of primary or

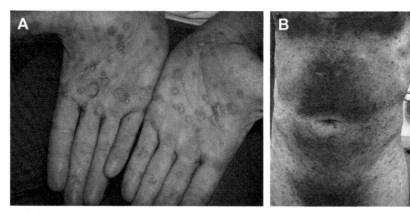

Fig. 6. (A) Palmar rash of secondary syphilis. (B) Truncal rash of secondary syphilis.

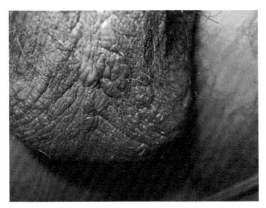

Fig. 7. Papulosquamous scrotal rash of secondary syphilis.

secondary syphilis; or (3) a sex partner documented to have primary, secondary, or early latent syphilis.[37]

Late Syphilis

Late latency is the asymptomatic phase of syphilis greater than 1 year after syphilis infection. Late latent syphilis, unlike early latent syphilis, is not thought to be infectious (except in pregnant women in whom transmission may occur), and requires a longer duration of treatment compared with early latent syphilis (see section on treatment).

Tertiary syphilis

Tertiary syphilis, or late symptomatic syphilis, has become very uncommon in the antibiotic era. In tertiary syphilis, endarteritis leads to cellular necrosis, fibrosis, sclerosis, scarring, and loss of normal tissue parenchyma. The three most common manifestations of tertiary disease are (1) neurologic; (2) cardiovascular; and (3) gummatous (or late benign) syphilis.

Late neurologic complications of syphilis As described previously, acute syphilitic meningitis can occur early in syphilis infection and is a well-described feature of secondary syphilis. Late neurologic complications of syphilis, which present after long periods of latency, are caused by meningovascular and/or parenchymal damage. Vascular involvement leading to focal ischemia can present with a myriad of neurologic deficits including hemiparesis, aphasia, and focal or generalized seizures.

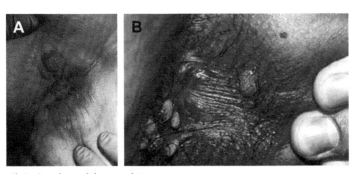

Fig. 8. (*A, B*) Perianal condylomata lata.

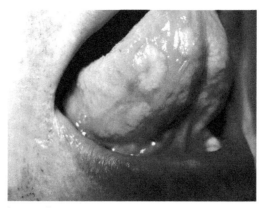

Fig. 9. Mucous patches on the tongue.

Classic late neurologic manifestations attributed to parenchymal damage include general paresis and tabes dorsalis.

General paresis, also known as general paralysis of the insane, is a meningoencephalitis with direct invasion of the cerebrum by *T pallidum*. The encephalitis is chronic and usually manifests in middle to late adulthood after a 15- to 20-year incubation period. A wide range of manifestations include progressive dementia with changes in personality, affect, sensorium, intellect, and speech. Defects in judgment, emotional lability, grandiose delusions, megalomania, depression, catatonia, amnesia, and hyperreflexia have been described. The Argyll Robertson pupil, a small, often irregularly shaped pupil that constricts on accommodation but not to light, is a classic though uncommon feature of general paresis.

Tabes dorsalis, syphilitic involvement of the posterior columns of the spinal cord, impacted about one-third of patients with late neurologic manifestations of syphilis in the preantibiotic era, but is now a very rare condition. The incubation period ranges from 20 to 25 years. Clinical symptoms include lightning pains, paresthesias, decreased reflexes, abnormalities in peripheral sensation, difficulty walking, and bladder and bowel dysfunction. Patients often have a positive Romberg sign. A classic description of tabes dorsalis includes patients who walk with their heels landing hard on the floor, knees positioned outward with their feet slapping.[36]

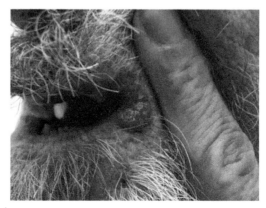

Fig. 10. Split papule.

Cardiovascular syphilis Endarteritis of the vaso vasorum of the aorta can lead to aortitis and aneurysm formation. This usually involves the ascending aorta, which in turn can cause dilation of the aortic ring, aortic regurgitation, or ascending aortic aneurysms.[8] Following the ascending aorta, the transverse aorta and then the descending arch are the next most common sites involved. Chronic inflammation of the coronary arteries can lead to narrowing and stenosis of the coronary ostia, which can ultimately lead to myocardial ischemia, infarction, and congestive heart failure.

Gummatous (or late benign) syphilis Gummatous disease is extremely uncommon and is characterized by indolent destructive lesions of the skin, soft tissue, and bony structures. Although those lesions are destructive, they respond rapidly to treatment. Visceral organs, bones, and the CNS can also be involved. The differential diagnosis of lesions of the skin and mucous membranes is broad and depends on the local epidemiology of other infectious diseases and neoplasms. Conditions to consider in the differential diagnosis of gummatous-appearing skin lesions include Hodgkin disease, mycosis fungoides, tuberculosis, systemic lupus erythematous, fungal infections, sarcoid, and granuloma annulare.

Congenital syphilis
The manifestations of congenital syphilis are variable and include asymptomatic disease, spontaneous abortion, intrauterine growth restriction, neonatal disease, and neonatal death. The fetus is usually infected transplacentally. Congenital infection is most likely to be acquired in the setting of maternal early syphilis; however, it has been documented at any stage of syphilis. Some of the classic features of neonatal disease include rhinitis (snuffles), which typically occurs early in the course of the disease, and rash, hepatitis, splenomegaly, and perichondritis or periostitis. Untreated neonates who survive neonatal syphilis enter a latent period. The perichondritis and periostitis can lead to deformities of the nose (saddle nose) and of the metaphyses of the lower extremities (saber shin). Other late manifestations of congenital syphilis include peg-shaped central incisors (Hutchinson teeth); frontal bossing; and recurrent arthropathy.[2,38]

Prevention and early detection of congenital syphilis depends on routine screening of pregnant women for syphilis. All pregnant women should be screened at the first prenatal visit. Women who are at high risk for syphilis infection should be screened again in the third trimester and at delivery (see diagnostic approach).[37]

DIAGNOSIS

Treponema pallidum cannot be cultivated in artificial media, is too slender to be observed by light microscopy, and fails to take up traditional Gram stains. It can be visualized using darkfield microscopy, which uses refracted light on a darkened background to identify the spirochete in clinical specimens; however, this technique is not widely available in clinical practice. Although polymerase chain reaction has been used to amplify genetic elements of *T pallidum* in clinical specimens, there are no current Food and Drug Administration cleared molecular amplification assays in use in routine clinical practice. The clinical diagnosis of syphilis is based on the characteristic findings of the skin and mucous membranes and is confirmed with serologic assays measuring antibodies to nontreponemal (rapid plasma reagin [RPR] or Venereal Disease Research Laboratory [VDRL] tests) and treponemal antigens (treponemal pallidum particle agglutination, fluorescent treponemal absorption, enzyme immunoassays [EIA], and chemiluminescence immunoassays).

Nontreponemal tests use a laboratory-prepared lecithin-cholesterol antigen to detect treponemal-directed antibody in the patient serum specimen. Nontreponemal tests have a sensitivity of approximately 86% in primary syphilis and 100% in secondary syphilis.[39] Nontreponemal tests are 98% specific, with false-positives associated with older age; autoimmune disease (eg, lupus); other infections (eg, bacterial endocarditis, rickettsial infection); chronic liver disease; intravenous drug use; and recent vaccination. Nontreponemal tests can be performed quantitatively and response to treatment is demonstrated by declining nontreponemal titers over time.

In traditional syphilis screening algorithms, treponemal-specific tests are used to confirm the diagnosis of syphilis and to rule out false-positives in the setting of a positive nontreponemal test. The fluorescent treponemal antibody absorbed (FTA-ABS), *T pallidum* particle agglutination (TPPA), and *T pallidum* hemagglutination assay use true treponemal antigens as a key reagent. Unlike nontreponemal antibody tests, which decline in titer with treatment, treponemal-specific tests typically remain reactive for the remainder of the life of the individual irrespective of the success of treatment. Like nontreponemal tests, their sensitivity is lower in primary disease, although they may become reactive before nontreponemal tests in the earliest stages of primary infection. They are 100% sensitive and 99% specific in secondary disease.[39] By law, diagnosing clinicians and laboratories in the United States are required to report reactive laboratory tests for syphilis (treponemal and nontreponemal) to public health authorities.

Some clinical laboratories and blood banks have begun to use a treponemal EIA in place of a nontreponemal assay as a more cost-effective initial screening test for syphilis. A positive treponemal EIA identifies persons with a history of treated syphilis and those with untreated or incompletely treated syphilis. If the treponemal EIA is positive, a nontreponemal test should be obtained to determine the titer for monitoring response to treatment. This is known as "reverse sequence screening." If the nontreponemal test is nonreactive, a second treponemal-specific antibody test (TPPA or FTA-ABS) should be obtained because the initial EIA result could be a false-positive.[37] Although the specificity of the available syphilis EIAs is generally high, the positive predictive value of the test depends on the prevalence of syphilis in the population being screened. In low-prevalence settings, up to 40% of EIA-positive, RPR-negative specimens may be false-positives.[40,41] If two treponemal-specific antibody tests are positive and the nontreponemal test is nonreactive, this could represent latent infection, a previously treated case or, less likely, very early syphilis infection. In that situation, providers should closely examine the patient for any signs of primary syphilis and attempt to document prior treatment; sexually transmitted disease control programs within local or state health departments can often assist in this effort. If that is not possible, the diagnosis and treatment of latent syphilis should be considered.

Primary Syphilis

Evaluation of a patient who presents with a genital ulcer should include (1) sexual, medical, and medication history; (2) oral, skin (trunk, upper and lower extremities, palms and soles, scrotum), genital, and anal examination; (3) darkfield microscopic examination of suspicious lesions if available (serous exudate from a chancre can be examined for the presence of spirochetes); (4) serum nontreponemal tests like the RPR or VDRL and treponemal tests like the TPPA or FTA-ABS (because treponemal-specific tests may be more sensitive in early disease); (5) herpes simplex virus culture or polymerase chain reaction in a swab of an ulcer; and (6) serology for HIV infection (particularly essential if syphilis is diagnosed).

Secondary Syphilis

A rash of any type in a sexually active individual should be considered as potential syphilis until proved otherwise, particularly if it is bilaterally symmetric. The typical rash of secondary syphilis does not yield moist specimens for darkfield examination; however, if condylomata lata are present, and darkfield microscopy is available, these can be swabbed and examined directly for spirochetes. Nontreponemal tests are highly sensitive in secondary syphilis. A prozone phenomenon can occur when the antitreponemal antibody titer is so high that the characteristic agglutination reaction that produces a reactive specimen cannot occur. When the clinical suspicion for secondary syphilis is high and the nontreponemal test is negative, the test should be repeated with additional dilutions, usually 1:10.

Tertiary Syphilis

Serologic tests are usually reactive in tertiary syphilis; titers of nontreponemal tests can range from low to very high titers, but are usually lower than in early syphilis. In patients with neurologic findings concerning for late neurosyphilis and positive serum nontreponemal and treponemal antibody tests, the CSF should be examined. In addition, the CSF should be examined in a patient diagnosed with any other form of tertiary syphilis (cardiovascular or gummatous). A positive CSF VDRL establishes the diagnosis of neurosyphilis.

CSF Analysis: Indications and Interpretation

Syphilis can involve the CNS at any stage of disease. Asymptomatic invasion of the CNS is common in early syphilis, and abnormalities of the CSF have been found in up to 40% of patients with untreated secondary syphilis.[36,42] The clinical significance of those findings is unclear, because most patients with early syphilis respond appropriately to standard therapy. The CSF should therefore be examined in any patient with syphilis and any neurologic or ophthalmic symptoms or signs (cognitive dysfunction, motor or sensory defects, visual or auditory symptoms, cranial nerve palsies, meningismus). A CSF examination should also be considered in patients who fail to respond to therapy with an appropriate decline in nontreponemal antibody titer.[37] Although CSF abnormalities are more common in HIV-infected persons with syphilis and RPR titers greater than or equal to 1:32 and/or CD4 T-cell counts less than or equal to 350 cells/mm^3, in the absence of neurologic symptoms, there is no evidence that CSF examination in such persons is associated with improved clinical outcomes.[43,44]

Lymphocytic pleocytosis (10–500 WBC/mm^3) and elevated CSF total protein are characteristic of the acute, syphilitic meningitis seen in early syphilis. Fewer cells are seen in the CSF in late neurosyphilis, including syphilitic cerebrovascular disease, general paresis, and tabes dorsalis. An absence of white blood cells in the CSF excludes the diagnosis of neurosyphilis. In the setting of a reactive serum nontreponemal and treponemal antibody test, a reactive CSF VDRL confirms the diagnosis of neurosyphilis. However, the CSF VDRL, particularly in early syphilitic meningitis, is not highly sensitive. The role of other serologic tests in the CSF is uncertain. The CSF FTA-ABS has a high false-positive rate, but is more sensitive than the CSF VDRL. The CSF FTA-ABS can be used to exclude neurosyphilis in at-risk patients with an abnormal CSF and a negative CSF VDRL.

Congenital Syphilis

The diagnosis of congenital syphilis rests on the identification of syphilis in the mother, and a combination of clinical, radiologic, and laboratory findings in the infant. All infants born to mothers with reactive nontreponemal and treponemal test results should be screened for congenital syphilis by performing a quantitative nontreponemal antibody test on infant serum (not umbilical cord blood, which can become contaminated with maternal blood). The infant should be examined carefully for signs and symptoms of syphilis. If clinically indicated, the work-up may include long-bone radiographs; chest radiograph; liver function tests; cranial ultrasound; ophthalmologic examination; auditory examination; and CSF analysis for VDRL, cell count, and protein.[2,37] The evaluation and management of congenital syphilis should be made in consultation with a pediatric infectious diseases specialist.

TREATMENT

Penicillin G remains the treatment of choice for all stages of syphilis. The treatment regimen (route of administration and duration) depends on the stage of disease (**Table 1**). Early syphilis (ie, primary, secondary, or early latent) can be treated with a single injection of 2.4 million units of intramuscular penicillin G benzathine; patients coinfected with HIV do not require additional doses of penicillin.[37,45–47] A nontreponemal antibody test should be obtained on the day of treatment to establish a baseline titer for monitoring response to therapy. Late syphilis (late latent syphilis and syphilis of unknown duration) is treated with penicillin G benzathine, 2.4 million units intramuscular weekly for a total of three injections given a week apart without missing any doses.[37,48] A lapse of more than 14 days requires restarting treatment. Neurosyphilis is treated with intravenous aqueous penicillin G, 2.4 million units every 4 hours for 10 to 14 days. Intravenous treatment should be followed by penicillin G benzathine, 2.4 million units intramuscularly weekly for 3 weeks. Patients with syphilitic uveitis or other ocular manifestations should be treated according to the recommendations for neurosyphilis.[37]

Approximately 10% of patients self-report a history of a penicillin allergy, but the rates of true penicillin allergy are likely much lower.[49] Other antibiotics have efficacy and can be used, if necessary, in the setting of penicillin allergy. Doxycycline is effective for early stage syphilis (100 mg orally twice daily for 14 days) and for late syphilis (100 mg orally twice daily for 28 days).[37,48,50] Daily ceftriaxone (1–2 g daily either IM or IV for 10–14 days) can be used as an alternative to penicillin,[51,52] and the risk of penicillin cross-reactivity with third-generation cephalosporins is negligible.[53] A randomized controlled trial conducted among HIV-uninfected patients outside the United States found that oral azithromycin administered at a dosage of 2 g was equivalent to benzathine penicillin G, 2.4 million units intramuscularly, for the treatment of early syphilis.[54] However, given documented cases of azithromycin treatment failures and evidence of *T pallidum* resistance to azithromycin in the United States, there is limited role for azithromycin in the treatment of syphilis in the United States.[55,56]

FOLLOW-UP

Patients with early stage syphilis, particularly those with high titer secondary syphilis, should be counseled about the possibility that they may experience a Jarisch-Herxheimer reaction after treatment. This immune-mediated process occurs within 2 to 24 hours of receiving penicillin G and is characterized by the acute onset of fever, headache, and myalgias. Peripheral leukocytosis and transaminitis can also occur. It occurs in 50% to 75% of patients with primary and secondary syphilis, is more common in patients with higher baseline nontreponemal titers, and is less common in patients with a history of treated syphilis.[57] The reaction is usually self-limited and can be managed with antipyretics and nonsteroidal anti-inflammatory medications. In pregnant women, the reaction may trigger preterm labor or other complications, so close monitoring in collaboration with the patient's obstetrician is essential, but this should not prevent or delay treatment.

Table 1
Treatment for syphilis

Syphilis Stage or Diagnosis	Primary Therapy	Alternative Therapy	Comment
Primary, secondary, and early latent syphilis	Penicillin G benzathine, 2.4 million units IM as a single dose	Doxycycline, 100 mg PO twice daily for 14 d Or Ceftriaxone, 1–2 g either IM or IV daily for 10–14 d Or Tetracycline, 100 mg PO four times daily for 14 d	—
Late latent syphilis	Penicillin G benzathine, 2.4 million units IM once weekly for 3 wk	Doxycycline, 100 mg PO twice daily for 28 d Or Tetracycline, 100 mg PO four times daily for 28 d	—
Neurosyphilis	Penicillin G aqueous, 18–24 million units IV daily (3–4 million units q 4 h or by continuous infusion) for 10–14 d	Procaine penicillin, 2.4 million units IM daily *plus* probenecid, 500 mg PO four times daily, both for 10–14 d Or Ceftriaxone, 2 g either IM or IV daily for 10–14 d	Follow-up treatment with 3 additional weekly injections of penicillin G benzathine, 2.4 million units IM
Tertiary syphilis (not neurosyphilis)	Penicillin G benzathine, 2.4 million units IM once weekly for 3 wk	—	Cerebrospinal fluid evaluation should be performed before therapy

The response to treatment should be assessed by the resolution of clinical manifestations and by the decline in nontreponemal antibody titers over time. Successful therapy is determined by a fourfold decline in the nontreponemal antibody test (eg, 1:32–1:8). When monitoring response to treatment, the same nontreponemal test (either RPR or VDRL) should be followed serially because of variation in nontreponemal antibody titer according to test type. Ideally, all patients with syphilis should have follow-up titers measured at 3, 6, 9, 12, and 24 months posttreatment. Titers can rise transiently in the first few weeks after treatment, so retesting before 3 months is not recommended.[58] In early stage syphilis a fourfold decline should occur within 6 to 12 months of treatment. In late syphilis this decline can take 12 to 24 months.

Across studies, between 15% and 27% of patients with early syphilis fail to achieve a fourfold decline in titer after 12 months, irrespective of HIV infection status.[43,45,59] In addition, some patients achieve a fourfold decline but continue to have a "high" titer (eg, 1:32). The biologic and clinical significance of a lack of decline in titer or persistent "high" titer despite fourfold decline are unclear. Those cases may be caused by syphilis reinfection or less likely treatment failure. Repeat syphilis infections are common,[60] and by following serial nontreponemal antibody titers, it is easier to distinguish reinfection from treatment failure. Because treatment failure may be the result of unrecognized CNS infection, CSF examination can be considered if a fourfold decline in titer is not observed within the expected interval. If the CSF is abnormal, the patient should be treated for neurosyphilis. If the CSF is normal, optimal treatment is unclear and some experts recommend that treatment be reinitiated with penicillin G benzathine, 2.4 million units weekly for 3 weeks.[37] In a study of 82 HIV-negative patients who failed to achieve a fourfold decline 6 months after treatment of primary syphilis, retreatment with one additional dose of penicillin G benzathine, 2.4 million units, led to a serologic cure in only 27%.[61]

Whether HIV-infected patients with syphilis have a slower decline in nontreponemal antibody titer than HIV-uninfected patients is unclear, because results have varied between studies.[45,46,62,63] Given the possibility of slower titer decline, most experts recommend following up asymptomatic HIV-infected patients for a full 12 months for early syphilis and 24 months for late latent syphilis before making a determination of treatment failure.

PREGNANCY AND CONGENITAL SYPHILIS

Pregnant women with syphilis who are allergic to penicillin should be desensitized and treated with penicillin according to the guidelines listed previously.[37] In pregnant women the Jarisch-Herxheimer reaction can precipitate uterine contractions, fetal distress, or premature labor; thus, pregnant women should be treated in a monitored setting.[2,64] Treatment of neonates with proved or probable congenital syphilis should be done in consultation with a pediatric infectious diseases specialist.

PUBLIC HEALTH RESPONSE: MANAGEMENT OF SEX PARTNERS

Providers can work together with local health departments to prevent the spread of syphilis. Presumptive and confirmed cases of syphilis should be reported within 1 working day of diagnosis. Staff in public health departments are then able to contact and notify sex partners, and provide testing and treatment as appropriate. Internet partner notification (ie, using email and chat room "handles" to notify partners) can augment syphilis case management and is an important tool in the modern syphilis epidemic.[65] For patients exposed to early syphilis within the past 3 months the proper management includes examination; nontreponemal testing (stat, if available); and immediate treatment with penicillin regardless of serologic test results. For patients exposed to early syphilis who are beyond the 3-month incubation period, treatment depends on clinical examination findings and serologic test results. Presumptive treatment of contacts based on exposure history is essential to prevent reinfection and control the spread of disease.

REFERENCES

1. Radolf J, Lukehart S. Pathogenic treponema: molecular and cellular biology. Norfolk (England): Caister Academic Press; 2006.
2. De Santis M, De Luca C, Mappa I, et al. Syphilis infection during pregnancy: fetal risks and clinical management. Infect Dis Obstet Gynecol 2012;1–5.
3. Genc M, Ledger WJ. Syphilis in pregnancy. Sex Transm Infect 2000;76:73–9.
4. Dorfman DH, Glaser JH. Congenital syphilis presenting in infants after the newborn period. N Engl J Med 1990;323:1299–302.
5. Chambers RW, Foley HT, Schmidt PJ. Transmission of syphilis by fresh blood components. Transfusion 1969;9:32–4.
6. Owusu-Ofori AK, Parry CM, Bates I. Transfusion-transmitted syphilis in teaching hospital, Ghana. Emerg Infect Dis 2011;17:2080–2.
7. Perkins HA, Busch MP. Transfusion-associated infections: 50 years of relentless challenges and remarkable progress. Transfusion 2010;50:2080–99.
8. Cotran R, Kumar V, Collins T. Robbins pathologic basis of disease. 6th edition. Philadelphia: W.B. Saunders Company; 1999.
9. Centers for Disease Control and Prevention. Sexually transmitted disease surveillance 2011. Atlanta (GA): U.S. Department of Health and Human Services; 2012.
10. Centers for Disease Control and Prevention. The National Plan to Eliminate syphilis from the United States. Atlanta (GA): U.S. Department of Health and Human Services; 1999.
11. Bernstein KT, Stephens SC, Strona FV, et al. Epidemiologic characteristics of an ongoing syphilis epidemic among men who have sex with men, San Francisco. Sex Transm Dis 2013;40:11–7.
12. Kerani RP, Handsfield HH, Stenger MS, et al. Rising rates of syphilis in the era of syphilis elimination. Sex Transm Dis 2007;34:154–61.
13. Zetola NM, Klausner JD. Syphilis and HIV infection: an update. Clin Infect Dis 2007;44:1222–8.
14. Phipps W, Kent CK, Kohn R, et al. Risk factors for repeat syphilis in men who have sex with men, San Francisco. Sex Transm Dis 2009;36:331–5.
15. Buchacz K, Klausner JD, Kerndt PR, et al. HIV incidence among men diagnosed with early syphilis in Atlanta, San Francisco, and Los Angeles, 2004 to 2005. J Acquir Immune Defic Syndr 2008;47:234–40.
16. Fenton KA. A multilevel approach to understanding the resurgence and evolution of infectious syphilis in Western Europe. Euro Surveill 2004;9:3–4.
17. Fenton KA, Breban R, Vardavas R, et al. Infectious syphilis in high-income settings in the 21st century. Lancet Infect Dis 2008;8:244–53.
18. Heffelfinger JD, Swint EB, Berman SM, et al. Trends in primary and secondary syphilis among men who have sex with men in the United States. Am J Public Health 2007;97:1076–83.
19. Wong W, Chaw JK, Kent CK, et al. Risk factors for early syphilis among gay and bisexual men seen in an STD clinic: San Francisco, 2002-2003. Sex Transm Dis 2005;32:458–63.

20. Jin F, Prestage GP, Kippax SC, et al. Epidemic syphilis among homosexually active men in Sydney. Med J Aust 2005;183:179–83.

21. Imrie J, Lambert N, Mercer CH, et al. Refocusing health promotion for syphilis prevention: results of a case-control study of men who have sex with men on England's south coast. Sex Transm Infect 2006;82:80–3.

22. Sullivan PS, Drake AJ, Sanchez TH. Prevalence of treatment optimism-related risk behavior and associated factors among men who have sex with men in 11 states, 2000-2001. AIDS Behav 2007;11:123–9.

23. Stolte IG, Dukers NH, Geskus RB, et al. Homosexual men change to risky sex when perceiving less threat of HIV/AIDS since availability of highly active antiretroviral therapy: a longitudinal study. AIDS 2004;18:303–9.

24. Internet use and early syphilis infection among men who have sex with men—San Francisco, California, 1999-2003. MMWR Morb Mortal Wkly Rep 2003;52: 1229–32.

25. Chesson HW, Gift TL. Decreases in AIDS mortality and increases in primary and secondary syphilis in men who have sex with men in the United States. J Acquir Immune Defic Syndr 2008;47:263–4.

26. Truong HM, Kellogg T, Klausner JD, et al. Increases in sexually transmitted infections and sexual risk behaviour without a concurrent increase in HIV incidence among men who have sex with men in San Francisco: a suggestion of HIV serosorting? Sex Transm Infect 2006;82:461–6.

27. Charlebois ED, Das M, Porco TC, et al. The effect of expanded antiretroviral treatment strategies on the HIV epidemic among men who have sex with men in San Francisco. Clin Infect Dis 2011;52:1046–9.

28. Raymond HF, Chen YH, Ick T, et al. A new trend in the HIV epidemic among men who have sex with men, San Francisco, 2004-2011. J Acquir Immune Defic Syndr 2013;62:584–9.

29. Schmid GP, Stoner BP, Hawkes S, et al. The need and plan for global elimination of congenital syphilis. Sex Transm Dis 2007;34:S5–10.

30. Chen ZQ, Zhang GC, Gong XD, et al. Syphilis in China: results of a national surveillance programme. Lancet 2007;369:132–8.

31. Tucker JD, Cohen MS. China's syphilis epidemic: epidemiology, proximate determinants of spread, and control responses. Curr Opin Infect Dis 2011;24:50–5.

32. Harrison LW. The Oslo study of untreated syphilis, review and commentary. Br J Vener Dis 1956;32:70–8.

33. Jones JH. Bad blood: the Tuskegee Syphilis experiment. 2nd edition. New York: Free Press; 1993.

34. Reverby SM. Normal exposure and inoculation syphilis: a PHS Tuskegee doctor in Guatemala, 1946-48. J Pol Hist 2011;23:6–28.

35. Presidential Commission for the Study of Bioethical Issues. "Ethically impossible" STD research in Guatemala from 1946 to 1948. Washington, DC: 2011. Available at: www.bioethics.gov.

36. Sparling PF, Swartz MN, Musher DM, et al. Sexually transmitted diseases. 4th edition. New York: McGraw Hill Medical; 2008.

37. Workowski KA, Berman S. Sexually transmitted diseases treatment guidelines, 2010. MMWR Recomm Rep 2010;59:1–110.

38. Walker GJ, Walker DG. Congenital syphilis: a continuing but neglected problem. Semin Fetal Neonatal Med 2007;12:198–206.

39. Sena AC, White BL, Sparling PF. Novel *Treponema pallidum* serologic tests: a paradigm shift in syphilis screening for the 21st century. Clin Infect Dis 2010; 51:700–8.

40. Discordant results from reverse sequence syphilis screening—five laboratories, United States, 2006-2010. MMWR Morb Mortal Wkly Rep 2011;60:133–7.
41. Park IU, Chow JM, Bolan G, et al. Screening for syphilis with the treponemal immunoassay: analysis of discordant serology results and implications for clinical management. J Infect Dis 2011;204:1297–304.
42. Lukehart SA, Hook EW III, Baker-Zander SA, et al. Invasion of the central nervous system by *Treponema pallidum*: implications for diagnosis and treatment. Ann Intern Med 1988;109:855–62.
43. Ghanem KG, Workowski KA. Management of adult syphilis. Clin Infect Dis 2011; 53(Suppl 3):S110–28.
44. Marra CM, Maxwell CL, Smith SL, et al. Cerebrospinal fluid abnormalities in patients with syphilis: association with clinical and laboratory features. J Infect Dis 2004;189:369–76.
45. Dionne-Odom J, Karita E, Kilembe W, et al. Syphilis treatment response among HIV-discordant couples in Zambia and Rwanda. Clin Infect Dis 2013;56: 1829–37.
46. Rolfs RT, Joesoef MR, Hendershot EF, et al. A randomized trial of enhanced therapy for early syphilis in patients with and without human immunodeficiency virus infection. The Syphilis and HIV Study Group. N Engl J Med 1997;337: 307–14.
47. Blank LJ, Rompalo AM, Erbelding EJ, et al. Treatment of syphilis in HIV-infected subjects: a systematic review of the literature. Sex Transm Infect 2011;87:9–16.
48. Wong T, Singh AE, De P. Primary syphilis: serological treatment response to doxycycline/tetracycline versus benzathine penicillin. Am J Med 2008;121: 903–8.
49. Park M, Markus P, Matesic D, et al. Safety and effectiveness of a preoperative allergy clinic in decreasing vancomycin use in patients with a history of penicillin allergy. Ann Allergy Asthma Immunol 2006;97:681–7.
50. Ghanem KG, Erbelding EJ, Cheng WW, et al. Doxycycline compared with benzathine penicillin for the treatment of early syphilis. Clin Infect Dis 2006;42: e45–9.
51. Hook EW III, Roddy RE, Handsfield HH. Ceftriaxone therapy for incubating and early syphilis. J Infect Dis 1988;158:881–4.
52. Psomas KC, Brun M, Causse A, et al. Efficacy of ceftriaxone and doxycycline in the treatment of early syphilis. Med Mal Infect 2012;42:15–9.
53. Pichichero ME, Casey JR. Safe use of selected cephalosporins in penicillin-allergic patients: a meta-analysis. Otolaryngol Head Neck Surg 2007;136: 340–7.
54. Hook EW III, Behets F, Van Damme K, et al. A phase III equivalence trial of azithromycin versus benzathine penicillin for treatment of early syphilis. J Infect Dis 2010;201:1729–35.
55. A2058G Prevalence Workgroup. Prevalence of the 23S rRNA A2058G point mutation and molecular subtypes in *Treponema pallidum* in the United States, 2007 to 2009. Sex Transm Dis 2012;39:794–8.
56. Katz KA, Klausner JD. Azithromycin resistance in *Treponema pallidum*. Curr Opin Infect Dis 2008;21:83–91.
57. Yang CJ, Lee NY, Lin YH, et al. Jarisch-Herxheimer reaction after penicillin therapy among patients with syphilis in the era of the HIV infection epidemic: incidence and risk factors. Clin Infect Dis 2010;51:976–9.
58. Holman KM, Wolff M, Sena AC, et al. Rapid plasma reagin titer variation in the 2 weeks after syphilis therapy. Sex Transm Dis 2012;39:645–7.

59. Sena AC, Wolff M, Martin DH, et al. Predictors of serological cure and serofast state after treatment in HIV-negative persons with early syphilis. Clin Infect Dis 2011;53:1092–9.
60. Cohen SE, Chew Ng RA, Katz KA, et al. Repeat syphilis among men who have sex with men in California, 2002-2006: implications for syphilis elimination efforts. Am J Public Health 2011;102:e1–8.
61. Sena AC, Wolff M, Behets F, et al. Response to therapy following retreatment of serofast early syphilis patients with benzathine penicillin. Clin Infect Dis 2013;56:420–2.
62. Knaute DF, Graf N, Lautenschlager S, et al. Serological response to treatment of syphilis according to disease stage and HIV status. Clin Infect Dis 2012;55:1615–22.
63. Gonzalez-Lopez JJ, Guerrero ML, Lujan R, et al. Factors determining serologic response to treatment in patients with syphilis. Clin Infect Dis 2009;49:1505–11.
64. Myles TD, Elam G, Park-Hwang E, et al. The Jarisch-Herxheimer reaction and fetal monitoring changes in pregnant women treated for syphilis. Obstet Gynecol 1998;92:859–64.
65. Ehlman DC, Jackson M, Saenz G, et al. Evaluation of an innovative internet-based partner notification program for early syphilis case management, Washington, DC, January 2007-June 2008. Sex Transm Dis 2010;37:478–85.

Control of *Neisseria gonorrhoeae* in the Era of Evolving Antimicrobial Resistance

Lindley A. Barbee, MD, MPH[a,b,]*, Julia C. Dombrowski, MD, MPH[a,b]

KEYWORDS

- *Neisseria gonorrhoeae* • Sexually transmitted disease • Antimicrobial resistance

KEY POINTS

- Gonorrhea is the second most common bacterial sexually transmitted disease worldwide. Untreated infection can lead to infertility in women, and increase the risk of transmission and acquisition of the human immunodeficiency virus.
- Cephalosporin-resistant *Neisseria gonorrhoeae* is now a major public health threat as strains demonstrating decreased susceptibility to oral cephalosporins become more common.
- Although a few ceftriaxone treatment failures have been reported worldwide, intramuscular ceftriaxone combined with oral azithromycin remains a highly effective treatment for gonorrhea.
- Screening for asymptomatic infections in women at risk and men who have sex with men is central to gonorrhea control.

INTRODUCTION

Gonorrhea is one of the most common curable sexually transmitted diseases (STDs), affecting more than 106 million individuals throughout the globe[1] and an estimated 700,000 individuals in the United States each year.[2] Gonorrhea disproportionately

Funding Sources: Dr L.A. Barbee: National Institutes of Health Sexually Transmitted Diseases Training Grant [T32 67-4198], National Institutes of Allergy and Infectious Diseases, Division of Microbiology and Infectious Diseases Contract #HHSN272200800026C, and the Seattle Sexually Transmitted Diseases Prevention Training Center; Dr J.C. Dombrowski: National Institutes of Mental Health (K23MH090923) and the University of Washington Center for AIDS Research (CFAR), an NIH funded program (P30 AI027757), which is supported by the following NIH Institutes and Centers: NIAID, NCI, NIMH, NIDA, NICHD, NHLBI, and NIA.
Conflicts of Interest: None.
[a] Department of Medicine, Division of Allergy and Infectious Diseases, Harborview Medical Center, University of Washington, Box 359777, 325 9th Avenue, Seattle, WA 98104, USA;
[b] HIV/STD Program, Public Health – Seattle & King County, 325 9th Avenue, Box 359777, Seattle, WA 98104, USA
* Corresponding author.
E-mail address: lbarbee@u.washington.edu

Infect Dis Clin N Am 27 (2013) 723–737
http://dx.doi.org/10.1016/j.idc.2013.08.001
0891-5520/13/$ – see front matter © 2013 Elsevier Inc. All rights reserved.

affects women, men who have sex with men (MSM), and racial/ethnic minorities. In women, untreated *Neisseria gonorrhoeae* infection can lead to major morbidities including pelvic inflammatory disease, ectopic pregnancy, tubal factor infertility, and congenital blindness in offspring.[3] In all persons, gonorrhea increases the risk of transmission and acquisition of the human immunodeficiency virus (HIV).[4] Although once one of public health's great success stories, gonorrhea is once again a major public health threat with the emergence of multidrug resistance.[5]

Epidemiology

Gonorrhea rates in the United States declined almost 80% from the mid-1970s to the late 1990s, after the introduction of a national gonorrhea control program. With those declines, rates of pelvic inflammatory disease and ectopic pregnancy plummeted.[3] However, in the United States since 2002, women have consistently had higher rates of gonorrhea than men. Gonorrhea rates are highest among young women aged 15 to 24 years, with 108.9 cases for every 100,000 women in 2011.[6] Racial/ethnic disparities in gonorrhea incidence are profound, with rates in African Americans 17-fold those in whites, and rates in American Indians and Hispanics 4.6-fold and 2.1-fold those in whites, respectively. Gonorrhea incidence also varies substantially by geography, with the highest rates in the United States found in southeastern states. Among a network of 12 sentinel STD surveillance sites nationwide, the distribution of gonococcal infections by gender and sexual orientation was 21.6% MSM, 31% heterosexual men, and 47.4% women, although the distribution varied widely by geographic region. For example, in San Francisco less than 10% of diagnosed gonococcal infections occurred in women, whereas in Alabama, Connecticut, and Virginia more than 60% of infections were in women.[6]

Worldwide, gonorrhea rates are increasing. The World Health Organization (WHO) estimates that gonorrhea cases increased 21% between 2005 and 2008, from 87 million to 106 million annual cases. Although the yearly incidence of gonorrhea is higher in men than women worldwide, women bear a larger burden of prevalent infections[1] attributable, in part, to the primarily asymptomatic nature of infections in women. The WHO regions of the Western Pacific (eg, China, Japan, the Philippines, Malaysia, Vietnam, Australia), Southeast Asia (eg, India, Korea, Thailand, Bangladesh), and Africa have the highest gonorrhea rates in the world.[1]

Antimicrobial Surveillance

The primary source for surveillance of antimicrobial resistance in gonorrhea in the United States is the Gonococcal Isolate Surveillance Project (GISP), a collaboration of 28 sentinel clinic sites and 5 regional laboratories funded by the Centers for Disease Control and Prevention (CDC). GISP was started in 1986 to provide an evidence base for the selection of gonococcal treatment.[7] Although GISP tests only urethral isolates from men diagnosed in STD clinics, the CDC STD Surveillance Network (SSuN) now has pilot programs for enhanced surveillance of extragenital gonorrhea isolates from MSM and isolates from patients with possible treatment failures (SSuN cooperative agreement info: CDC-RFA-PS08-865).

The WHO Gonococcal Antimicrobial Surveillance Program (GASP) was introduced in 1992 to monitor antimicrobial resistance in *N gonorrhoeae* in the Western Pacific Region. GASP was expanded in 2007/2008 with the addition of the South East Asia Region.[8] In Europe, antimicrobial surveillance is performed by Euro-GASP, which was created in 2004 as part of the European Surveillance of Sexually Transmitted Infections and continues today through the European Center for Disease Prevention and Control.[9]

EVOLUTION OF ANTIMICROBIAL RESISTANCE IN *NEISSERIA GONORRHOEAE*

N gonorrhoeae is adept at acquiring antimicrobial resistance, and the effort to stay ahead of gonococcal evolution has defined its treatment since the inception of antibiotics. The WHO recommends removing an antibiotic from first-line therapy recommendations for treatment of an STD when more than 5% of isolates in a community are resistant to the antibiotic.[10] Although there are no empirical data to support a particular threshold, the 5% mark has been influential in the formation of STD treatment guidelines. Sulfonamides, developed in the 1930s, were one of the first widely used classes of antibiotics, but had a relatively short life as gonococcal therapy because resistance emerged within 10 years of their introduction. By the mid-1940s, penicillin had become the mainstay of gonococcal treatment. Penicillin was a remarkably resilient therapy, but over the course of 4 decades the minimum inhibitory concentration (MIC) of penicillin in *N gonorrhoeae* gradually rose along with the recommended dose of penicillin for gonorrhea treatment. By the late 1980s, penicillin ceased to be an adequate treatment. Nearly simultaneously, resistance to tetracyclines, an alternative therapy, also emerged.[10] Fortunately, at that time alternative drug classes were available.

Third-generation cephalosporins and quinolones became the recommended therapies in the late 1980s. However, resistance to quinolones emerged rapidly, originally in East and Southeast Asia. By the mid-1990s quinolone-resistant gonorrhea was detected in North America, initially in Hawaii, and then on the West coast of the United States[10] By 2006, 39% of gonorrhea isolates from MSM in the United States were quinolone resistant, and quinolones were removed from the CDC gonorrhea treatment guidelines.[11] Since 2006, the CDC has recommended only one class of antimicrobials as a first-line therapy for gonorrhea: the cephalosporins. Following the historical pattern witnessed with quinolone resistance, the gonococcus is now developing resistance to cephalosporins as well.

Contemporary Cephalosporin Resistance

To date, there is no universal laboratory definition of gonorrhea resistance to cephalosporins (**Table 1**). MIC breakpoints for decreased susceptibility differ for cefixime, an oral third-generation cephalosporin, and ceftriaxone, a parenteral third-generation

Table 1 Comparative definitions of minimum inhibitory concentration (MIC) breakpoints for decreased susceptibility to selected antibiotics and MICs of isolates reported as "superbugs"			
	Cefixime MIC (µg/mL)	Ceftriaxone MIC (µg/mL)	Azithromycin MIC (µg/mL)
CLSI: decreased susceptibility	≥0.5	≥0.5	NA
CDC alert value	≥0.25	≥0.125	≥2[a]
EUCAST: decreased susceptibility	≥0.25	≥0.25	≥1
WHO: decreased susceptibility	≥0.25	≥0.125	NA
Japanese isolate H041	8	2[b]	1
French isolate F89	4	1	1

Abbreviations: CDC, US Centers for Disease Control and Prevention; CLSI, US Clinical Laboratory Standards Institute; EUCAST, The European Committee on Antimicrobial Susceptibility Testing; NA, no data available; WHO, World Health Organization.

[a] CLSI does not define azithromycin resistance, but CDC uses 2 µg/mL to indicated decreased susceptibility.

[b] 2 µg/mL by agar dilution method, 4 µg/mL by e-test method.

cephalosporin. Similarly, terminology related to antimicrobial resistance varies. For instance, the US Clinical and Laboratory Standards Institute (CLSI) defines decreased susceptibility for both cefixime and ceftriaxone as an MIC of 0.5 μg/mL or higher,[12] whereas the CDC defines an "alert value" for cefixime as an MIC of 0.25 μg/mL or higher and an alert value for ceftriaxone as an MIC of 0.125 μg/mL or higher.[12]

Decreased cephalosporin susceptibility first emerged among gonorrhea strains in Asia. In Japan, between 1999 and 2002 the percentage of N gonorrhoeae isolates with an MIC to cefixime of 0.5 μg/mL or greater increased from zero to 30%.[13] Reports from Hong Kong and South Korea also documented increasing cephalosporin resistance,[14,15] and the WHO GASP for the Western Pacific and South-East Asia found at least 1 country in the region with 56% of its tested isolates exhibiting decreased susceptibility to ceftriaxone,[16] suggesting a larger pattern of emerging resistance throughout Asia.

In the United States, the proportion of gonorrhea isolates with CDC-designated cefixime alert-value MIC increased from 0.1% in 2006 to 1.7% in the first 6 months of 2011 (**Fig. 1**).[5] Although the proportion of isolates meeting the CLSI definition for decreased susceptibility to cefixime (≥0.5 μg/mL) also rose, these isolates accounted for only 0.1% of all isolates tested in 2006 to 2011. Of note, 77% of the isolates with elevated MICs to cefixime during this time were resistant to tetracycline.[12] Between 2006 and 2011 the proportion of tested isolates with alert-value MICs for ceftriaxone (≥0.125 μg/mL) rose from 0% to 0.4%.[12] Recapitulating the pattern observed in the spread of quinolone-resistant gonorrhea, decreased susceptibility strains are disproportionately found among MSM on the west coast of the United States.[5]

Using the European Committee on Antimicrobial Susceptibility Testing (EUCAST) criteria for decreased susceptibility to cefixime, 9% of isolates tested in Europe in 2010 showed decreased susceptibility to cefixime (MIC ≥0.25 μg/mL). Many countries in Europe, including Germany, Spain, Italy, Greece, Norway, Sweden, and Slovakia, report that more than 5% of all isolates from 2010 through 2012 had decreased susceptibility to cefixime.[17] In Austria, Denmark, and Slovenia, more than 20% of isolates had reduced susceptibility to cefixime. However, in 2010 the European CDC did not find any isolates with decreased susceptibility to ceftriaxone.[18] In contrast to North American epidemiology, the majority of isolates with decreased susceptibility to cefixime in Europe occur in heterosexual men.

Cephalosporin Treatment Failures

The clinical correlates of cephalosporin MIC values in gonorrhea are not known, but treatment failures to both cefixime and ceftriaxone in persons infected with reduced-susceptibility isolates have been reported. The first reported treatment failures to oral cephalosporins occurred in Japan in the early 2000s in patients treated with multiple doses of 200 mg cefixime against isolates exhibiting MICs ranging from 0.125 μg/mL to 1 μg/mL.[19,20] The Japanese authorities responded quickly and transitioned to ceftriaxone as first-line treatment for gonorrhea in 2006.[21] In 2010, the first 2 cases of cefixime treatment failure in Europe were reported in heterosexual men in Norway, both of whom failed treatment with 400 mg of cefixime, but were cured with 500 mg of intramuscular ceftriaxone.[22] Cefixime treatment failures were then documented in England,[23] Austria,[24] France,[25] and Canada.[26] In contrast to previous reports, the gonorrhea strains isolated from the Canadian series of 9 patients with treatment failures all had cefixime MICs of 0.12 μg/mL or lower[26]: at least 1 dilution below the CLSI and EUCAST designated elevated MIC level.

Ceftriaxone treatment failures were heralded by a 2011 case report of pharyngeal gonorrhea in a female sex worker in Kyoto, Japan. The infecting strain, named H041,

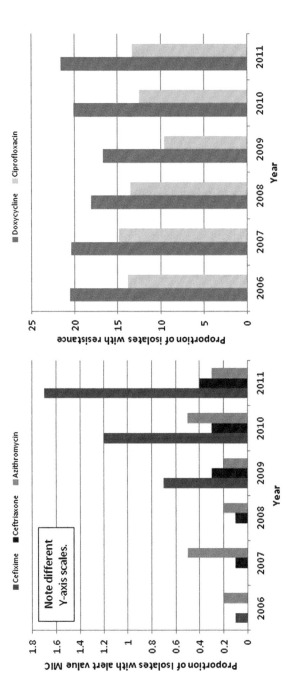

Fig. 1. Proportion of gonococcal isolates tested by GISP with CDC alert-value minimum inhibitory concentration (MIC) of cefixime, ceftriaxone, and azithromycin, and with resistance to doxycycline and ciprofloxacin: 2006 to August 2011. CDC defines alert-value MIC of cefixime as $\geq$0.25 µg/mL, ceftriaxone $\geq$0.125 µg/mL, and azithromycin $\geq$2.0 µg/mL. CDC defines doxycycline resistance as MIC $\geq$2.0 µg/mL and ciprofloxacin resistance as $\geq$1.0 µg/mL. Cefixime MIC was not tested in 2007 and 2008. (*Data from* CDC STD Surveillance Reports, 2006–2011.)

had a ceftriaxone MIC of 2 μg/mL, and was called the "superbug" because it also has high-level resistance to cefixime, penicillin, and levofloxacin.[27] Subsequently, ceftriaxone treatment failures were reported from Sweden,[28] Slovenia,[29] France,[25] and Spain.[30] The French isolate, F89, is considered the second strain of the gonococcal superbug, because of its resistance to cefixime, ceftriaxone, ciprofloxacin, azithromycin, tetracycline, and penicillin.[25] Although cases of ceftriaxone treatment failure have been rare to date, they are particularly concerning because they indicate the possibility of widespread, high-level cephalosporin resistance, leading to speculation about the possibility of an era of untreatable gonorrhea.

Molecular Mechanisms of Resistance

N gonorrhoeae has developed resistance to antimicrobials over time primarily because of its ability to scavenge DNA of other Neisseria species and incorporate exogenous DNA into its own genome (transformation). The gonococcus also develops resistance through acquisition of plasmids from other bacteria (conjugation), and spontaneous point mutations in response to antibiotic pressure.[31]

Three main resistance mutations result in decreased susceptibility to β-lactams: penA, mtrR, and penB. penA encodes a change in penicillin-binding protein 2 (PBP2), the primary site for β-lactams' mechanism of action. mtrR causes an efflux pump to be overexpressed, which leads to increased efflux of antibiotics, particularly ceftriaxone, and can also stimulate penB resistance mutation. penB alters the outermembrane porin (porB1b) to prevent cephalosporins from entering the cell. One potential explanation for the greater prevalence of cefixime resistance than ceftriaxone resistance among gonorrhea is that although nearly all cefixime resistance is due to the mosaic penA allele, ceftriaxone requires penA, mtrR, and penB mutations to result in clinically relevant resistance.[21,31,32]

SCREENING AND DIAGNOSIS

Gonorrhea can infect multiple mucosal surfaces, including urethral, cervicovaginal, oropharyngeal, rectal, and conjunctival sites. In men, urethral gonorrhea is almost always symptomatic. By contrast, at least 80% of women infected with gonorrhea will not exhibit symptoms.[3] For this reason, screening of asymptomatic women and partner treatment of heterosexual men with urethral infection are the cornerstones of gonorrhea control in women. In MSM, although 25% to 30% of urethral cases occur with concurrent pharyngeal infection,[33–36] the majority of all gonococcal infections in MSM are isolated to extragenital sites, the pharynx and/or rectum.[37] Extragenital infections are overwhelmingly asymptomatic[38] and underdiagnosed. The persistence of asymptomatic extragenital gonococcal infections in a community provides an important reservoir for ongoing transmission.

Screening Recommendations

The CDC recommends that all sexually active women younger than 25 years undergo annual screening for gonorrhea, and all pregnant women be screened in the first trimester with either a urine, vaginal, or endocervical nucleic acid amplification test (NAAT) (**Box 1**). Routine screening is also recommended for women older than 25 years who are at high risk for infection (eg, with multiple partners, previous history of STD, commercial sex worker, or part of a population with high prevalence of disease).[39] CDC guidelines recommend gonorrhea screening for all sexually active MSM annually with urine NAAT if they report insertive anal or oral intercourse, at the rectum if they report receptive anal intercourse, and at the pharynx if they report

---

Box 1
Screening recommendations

- All women younger than 25 years should be screened annually with urine or vaginal NAAT.

- Women older than 25 years at high risk for gonorrhea (eg, commercial sex work, multiple partners, a population with high prevalence of disease) should also routinely screen.

- All pregnant women should be screened during their first trimester.

- All MSM should be screened at least annually at all sites exposed in the last 12 months with NAAT (urethra, rectum, pharynx).

- MSM at high risk of infection (>10 partners per year, bacterial STD in prior 12 months, use amphetamines or amyl nitrates, unprotected anal intercourse) should screen as frequently as every 3 months.

Abbreviations: MSM, men who have sex with men; NAAT, nucleic acid amplification test; STD, sexually transmitted disease.

---

performing oral sex. Men who are at high risk of STDs, defined in the CDC guidelines as having multiple or anonymous partners, having had bacterial STD in the previous year, or users of methamphetamine or amyl nitrate, should be screened every 3 to 6 months.[39]

Screening of the pharynx and rectum is of utmost importance in MSM. Between 36% and 85% of gonorrhea infections in MSM are missed by urethral testing alone.[37,38] The data on screening for women for extragenital infection is mixed. Studies conducted in the 1970s and 1980s found that among women with genital tract infections with *N gonorrhoeae*, approximately 10% to 25% had concurrent pharyngeal gonorrhea,[33–36,40–42] and nearly 40% had concurrent rectal infection.[42] However, isolated extragenital infections (without concurrent cervical infection) in women were not common in those studies, and the US CDC does not recommend extragenital screening for women.[42–45] However, recent studies showing higher rates of extragenital coinfection have stimulated interest in revisiting extragenital screening recommendations for women.[43,46]

Diagnostic Technology

The advent of NAATs, which detect DNA or RNA, has changed the face of gonorrhea screening dramatically. Previous to the widespread use of NAATs, gonorrhea was diagnosed either in the clinic with a Gram stain of infected fluid or with culture. Culture is insensitive (50%–70% sensitivity)[3] but highly specific for the detection of gonorrhea. NAATs, on the other hand, are both highly sensitive and specific, and can be used to screen genital sites, urine, or other mucosal areas such as the throat and rectum. Because NAATs can detect nonviable genetic material, transportation and storage of specimens is less cumbersome than with culture, allowing for specimen collection at nonclinical venues. Although the Food and Drug Administration has yet to approve the use of NAATs on extragenital sites, many studies that have examined the performance of NAATs on pharyngeal and rectal specimens have validated their use,[47–49] and the US CDC now recommends the use of NAAT for extragenital screening.[39]

While the uptake of NAAT for gonorrhea testing is a positive step for gonorrhea control, the major drawback to this technology is the loss of widespread antimicrobial susceptibility testing. Assays designed to detect molecular markers of cephalosporin resistance in gonorrhea are under study, but are not commercially available or in widespread use.[50] Culture and antimicrobial susceptibility testing is not widely available outside of sites that participate in GISP and GASP, but clinicians who suspect a possible treatment failure should contact local public health authorities for assistance in arranging for culture-based testing.

Specimen Collection

Because NAATs require minimal technique for specimen collection, the type of specimen collection is more flexible than with culture. Since the introduction of NAATs, vaginal swabs have become the preferred specimen for gonococcal screening in women because of their superior sensitivity, although urine and cervical specimens are also highly sensitive.[51] In a study comparing first-void urine, self-collected vaginal specimens, and clinician-collected endocervical specimens, vaginal swabs yielded higher rates of gonorrhea detection than the other 2 methods.[52]

Another promising use of NAATs is for patient-collected specimens. Self-obtained testing facilitates screening in nonclinical settings, such as in the home or at outreach sites. Programs that offer home-based self-collected vaginal swabs increase testing volume[53] and case finding,[54] and successfully reach populations at risk.[53–56] Using the Aptima Combo 2, self-collected vaginal swabs perform comparably (sensitivity 98.7%, specificity 99.6%) with clinician-collected vaginal swabs (sensitivity 96.2%, specificity 99.4%).[51] Patients find self-collected vaginal swabs acceptable,[57] and most women prefer self-collection to a speculum examination or urine collection.[55,56]

Self-collection of extragenital specimens in MSM performs comparatively with, if not better than, clinician-obtained specimens.[58–60] In a study of 480 MSM, the concordance between self-collected and clinician-collected pharyngeal specimens for gonorrhea was 96.6%.[58] Concordance between rectal self-testing and clinician testing was 97.1% in another study.[60] Moreover, self-collection of extragenital specimens is acceptable to MSM, and when given a choice for asymptomatic screening, some MSM may prefer home-based testing.[61]

TREATMENT
Current Treatment Guidelines

The current treatment recommended by the US CDC for all uncomplicated gonococcal infections is 2-drug combination therapy with ceftriaxone 250 mg intramuscularly, and either azithromycin 1 g orally once or doxycycline 100 mg orally twice daily for 7 days (**Box 2**).[12,39] A single oral 400-mg dose of cefixime in combination with azithromycin

---

Box 2
Current CDC treatment guidelines

- For all uncomplicated gonococcal infections:

  Ceftriaxone 250 mg intramuscularly

  PLUS

  Azithromycin 1 g orally once OR doxycycline 100 mg orally twice daily for 7 days

- If ceftriaxone is not available, 400 mg cefixime orally once plus either azithromycin or doxycycline can be considered an alternative therapy, except for pharyngeal gonorrhea.

- Penicillin- or cephalosporin-allergic patients may be treated with 2 g azithromycin orally once.

- Persons treated with a nonceftriaxone containing regimen should return for a test-of-cure 7 to 10 days following therapy.

- All persons with gonococcal infection should return for rescreening 3 months following treatment.

or doxycycline has recently been downgraded to an alternative treatment reserved for uncomplicated urogenital infections.[12] Cefixime's removal from first-line treatment recommendations was based on the increasing proportion of isolates with alert-value MICs,[5] reports of treatment failures,[22–25] and its inadequacy in eradicating pharyngeal infections[39,62] that are often undiagnosed.[63,64] Highly effective treatment of pharyngeal gonorrhea is a priority, because untreated gonococcal infection in the oropharynx may contribute to sustained community transmission and promote the emergence of antimicrobial resistance arising from acquisition of resistance genes from commensal *Neisseria* species.[21,64]

The decision to recommend dual therapy was largely based on expert opinion, experience with other multidrug-resistant organisms whereby 2 or more drug regimens more effectively eradicate infection than single-drug regimens, and the theory that using 2 drugs may diminish the risk of inducing or selecting for resistance.[10,65] In practice, dual therapy for gonorrhea has been given for years as empiric cotreatment of chlamydial infections. Limited observational data support the rationale to move to dual therapy. Two retrospective studies suggest that treatment with cefixime and azithromycin is comparable with treatment with ceftriaxone, and superior to oral cephalosporin therapy alone or in combination with doxycycline for pharyngeal gonorrhea.[66,67]

Some nations have elected to increase the recommended dose of their chosen cephalosporin for gonorrhea treatment in an effort to combat emerging resistance. STD treatment guidelines in the United Kingdom recommend ceftriaxone 500 mg intramuscularly plus azithromycin 1 g.[68] Chinese and Japanese guidelines recommend 1 g ceftriaxone,[21] and Canadian guidelines recommend cefixime 800 mg once for most uncomplicated gonococcal infections, but prefer ceftriaxone 250 mg for MSM and pharyngeal infections.[69]

Potential Future Treatment Options

At present, there is only one novel drug approaching the clinical-trial stage for the treatment of cephalosporin-resistant gonorrhea. Solithromycin is an oral fluoroketolide, a form of a macrolide, which functions by binding to 3 binding sites on the bacterial ribosome. In vitro studies have found that solithromycin has good activity against cephalosporin-resistant gonorrhea, and against some isolates with low-level azithromycin resistance.[21,70] Furthermore, it has in vitro activity against *Chlamydia trachomatis* and *Mycoplasma genitalium*,[70,71] broadening its potential applicability in STD treatment.

Other options for the treatment of resistant gonorrhea include increasing the dose and duration of cephalosporins, reviving the use of older antibiotics, creating new combinations of antibiotics, and changing the tradition of STD treatment from empiric treatment to antimicrobial susceptibility–guided therapy for those with asymptomatic infections. Unemo and colleagues[72] reported that, among gonorrhea isolates with "resistant" level MICs to ceftriaxone ($\geq$0.5 μg/mL), the ertapenem MICs were much lower, suggesting that ertapenem could function as a backup regimen for ceftriaxone-resistant gonorrhea. Spectinomycin, not currently available in the United States, remains an option for uncomplicated anogenital gonococcal infection.[10] However, spectinomycin is not efficacious at eradicating gonorrhea from the pharynx, and resistance can emerge rapidly from a single point mutation.[21] Gentamicin has been used successfully as a single agent in practice in Malawi for years without the emergence of resistance,[21,73] but a meta-analysis found that gentamicin did not reach the prespecified population level of effectiveness (>95%) to warrant recommending its use for gonorrhea treatment.[74] Gemifloxacin is a fluoroquinolone with perseved in vitro activity against gonorrhea with ciprofloxacin resistance. The results of a clinical trial evaluating combination therapy with gemifloxacin (320 mg orally) plus azithromycin

(2 g orally) compared with azithromycin (2 g orally) plus gentamicin (240 mg intramuscularly) demonstrated high microbiological cure rates with both regimens (99.5% and 98.5%, respectively).[75]

Test-of-Cure and Rescreening

Test-of-cure, a repeat test after gonorrhea treatment, is intended to detect treatment failures and is typically done 1 to 4 weeks following treatment. By contrast, rescreening is intended to detect reinfection after successful treatment and is recommended 3 months following treatment for all persons diagnosed with gonorrhea, owing to the high risk of reinfection.[76] In practice, less than half of persons treated for gonorrhea complete rescreening. Before the revised gonorrhea treatment guidelines in late 2012, tests-of-cure were reserved for pregnant women, persons who did not complete recommended therapy, and persons with persistent symptoms. Current guidelines recommend test-of-cure for all persons with gonorrhea 7 to 10 days after treatment if they are not treated with a ceftriaxone-containing regimen.[12] Although culture is preferable for distinguishing active infection from residual DNA of a successfully treated infection, CDC guidelines consider a positive NAAT 7 days posttreatment to represent a clinical failure.

GISP represents another mechanism to monitor for possible treatment failures. GISP laboratories notify ordering providers and health departments when an isolate with an elevated MIC to cefixime is detected. In such cases, the clinicians and health department should coordinate efforts to contact the patient for retesting at all exposed sites and treatment with first-line therapy, and trace partners to ensure that all partners are tested and treated with a regimen containing ceftriaxone.[7,77]

Partner Treatment

Testing and treatment of sexual contacts is a central aspect of gonorrhea control. In all US states, clinicians are legally required to report cases of gonorrhea, and all sexual partners from the past 60 days should receive screening and empiric treatment. Expedited partner therapy (EPT), whereby patients deliver appropriate treatment directly to their sexual partners, increases partner treatment completion and reduces the likelihood of patients testing gonorrhea positive at follow-up.[78] Legal regulations regarding EPT vary by state, and EPT is not generally recommended for MSM owing to the high rates of undiagnosed HIV and STD coinfections in partners of men with gonorrhea. The CDC Cephalosporin-Resistant Neisseria gonorrhoeae Public Health Response Plan[77] recommends that persons exposed to gonorrhea be informed that dual therapy with ceftriaxone is the most effective treatment and be advised to seek clinical evaluation. However, EPT with cefixime and azithromycin is still an option encouraged for partner treatment of heterosexuals with gonorrhea in many states.[12,77] The potential for poorer treatment efficacy of decreased susceptibility gonorrhea isolates with a fully oral EPT regimen in sex partners of persons with gonorrhea must be considered in the context of higher treatment completion with EPT. Not all contacts to gonorrhea have gonococcal infection, and reduced susceptibility to cefixime in gonorrhea isolates from heterosexual men remains very rare.[77] Thus, at least at present, the public health benefits of EPT likely outweigh the risk of EPT-associated treatment failure.

A Gonorrhea Vaccine?

The ultimate solution for public health prevention of infectious disease is a vaccine. Unfortunately, efforts to develop a vaccine against gonorrhea have been met with many challenges. The primary challenge is the lack of sustained, systemic host immunity to gonorrhea. The immune response to gonococcal infections primarily occurs locally at the mucosal level. This local immunity is not sustained; hence, individuals may be reinfected multiple times with the same strain. At the level of the organism the gonococcal surface exhibits a variety of antigens, which can change over time, making identification of an antibody target difficult. Despite these impediments, investigators have made successful early steps toward a gonococcal vaccine.[21,79]

SUMMARY

Gonorrhea remains an important communicable disease across the globe, and the gonococcus' continual evolution to evade antimicrobials combined with a current lack of novel antimicrobial therapies makes cephalosporin-resistant gonorrhea a major public health threat. Increased screening of persons at risk for gonorrhea, appropriate and timely treatment of infected persons and their partners, active surveillance for antimicrobial resistance, and mobilization of public health resources in response to suspected cases of treatment failure are crucial for the control of cephalosporin-resistant gonorrhea.

REFERENCES

1. WHO. Global incidence and prevalence of selected curable sexually transmitted infections—2008. Geneva (Switzerland): World Health Organization; 2012.
2. CDC. Sexually transmitted disease surveillance, 2010. Atlanta (GA): US Department of Health and Human Services; 2011.
3. Marrazzo JM, Handsfield H, Sparling F. "Neisseria Gonorrhoeae". In: Mandell GL, Bennett JE, Dolin R, editors. Mandell, Douglas and Bennett's Principles and Practice of Infectious Diseases. 7th Edition. Philadelphia (PA): Elsevier; 2010.
4. Fleming DT, Wasserheit JN. From epidemiological synergy to public health policy and practice: the contribution of other sexually transmitted diseases to sexual transmission of HIV infection. Sex Transm Infect 1999;75(1):3–17.
5. Bolan GA, Sparling PF, Wasserheit JN. The emerging threat of untreatable gonococcal infection. N Engl J Med 2012;366(6):485–7.
6. CDC. Sexually transmitted disease surveillance, 2011. Atlanta (GA): US Department of Health and Human Services; 2012.
7. Kirkcaldy RD, Zaidi A, Hook EW, et al. *Neisseria gonorrhoeae* antimicrobial resistance among men who have sex with men and men who have sex exclusively with women: the gonococcal isolate surveillance project, 2005-2010. Ann Intern Med 2013;158(5 Pt 1):321–8.
8. Tapsall JW, Limnios EA, Abu Bakar HM, et al. Surveillance of antibiotic resistance in *Neisseria gonorrhoeae* in the WHO Western Pacific and South East Asian regions, 2007-2008. Commun Dis Intell 2010;34(1):1–7.
9. Cole MJ, Unemo M, Hoffmann S, et al. The European gonococcal antimicrobial surveillance programme, 2009. Euro Surveill 2011;16(42). pii: 19995.
10. Workowski KA, Berman SM, Douglas JM Jr. Emerging antimicrobial resistance in *Neisseria gonorrhoeae*: urgent need to strengthen prevention strategies. Ann Intern Med 2008;148(8):606–13.
11. Workowski KA, Berman SM. Sexually transmitted diseases treatment guidelines, 2006. MMWR Recomm Rep 2006;55(RR-11):1–94.
12. Centers for Disease Control and Prevention (CDC). Update to CDC's sexually transmitted diseases treatment guidelines, 2010: oral cephalosporins no longer a recommended treatment for gonococcal infections. MMWR Morb Mortal Wkly Rep 2012;61(31):590–4.

13. Ito M, Yasuda M, Yokoi S, et al. Remarkable increase in central Japan in 2001-2002 of *Neisseria gonorrhoeae* isolates with decreased susceptibility to penicillin, tetracycline, oral cephalosporins, and fluoroquinolones. Antimicrobial Agents Chemother 2004;48(8):3185–7.

14. Lo JY, Ho KM, Leung AO, et al. Ceftibuten resistance and treatment failure of *Neisseria gonorrhoeae* infection. Antimicrobial Agents Chemother 2008; 52(10):3564–7.

15. Lee H, Hong SG, Soe Y, et al. Trends in antimicrobial resistance of *Neisseria gonorrhoeae* isolated from Korean patients from 2000 to 2006. Sex Transm Dis 2011;38(11):1082–6.

16. Lahra MM. Surveillance of antibiotic resistance in *Neisseria gonorrhoeae* in the WHO Western Pacific and South East Asian Regions, 2010. Commun Dis Intell 2012;36(1):95–100.

17. Van de Laar M, Spiteri G. Increasing trends of gonorrhoea and syphilis and the threat of drug-resistant gonorrhoea in Europe. Euro Surveill 2012;17(29). pii: 20225.

18. European Centre for Disease Prevention and Control. Gonococcal antimicrobial susceptibility surveillance in Europe—2010. Stockholm (Sweden): European Centre for Disease Prevention and Control; 2012.

19. Yokoi S, Deguchi T, Ozawa T, et al. Threat to cefixime treatment for gonorrhea. Emerg Infect Dis 2007;13(8):1275–7.

20. Deguchi T, Yasuda M, Yokoi S, et al. Treatment of uncomplicated gonococcal urethritis by double-dosing of 200 mg cefixime at a 6-h interval. J Infect Chemother 2003;9(1):35–9.

21. Unemo M, Nicholas RA. Emergence of multidrug-resistant, extensively drug-resistant and untreatable gonorrhea. Future Microbiol 2012;7:1401–22.

22. Unemo M, Golparian D, Syversen G, et al. Two cases of verified clinical failures using internationally recommended first-line cefixime for gonorrhoea treatment, Norway, 2010. Euro Surveill 2010;15(47). pii: 19721.

23. Ison CA, Hussey J, Sankar KN, et al. Gonorrhoea treatment failures to cefixime and azithromycin in England, 2010. Euro Surveill 2011;16(14). pii: 19833.

24. Unemo M, Golparian D, Stary A, et al. First *Neisseria gonorrhoeae* strain with resistance to cefixime causing gonorrhoea treatment failure in Austria, 2011. Euro Surveill 2011;16(43). pii:19998.

25. Unemo M, Golparian D, Nicholas R, et al. High-level cefixime- and ceftriaxone-resistant *Neisseria gonorrhoeae* in France: novel penA mosaic allele in a successful international clone causes treatment failure. Antimicrobial Agents Chemother 2012;56(3):1273–80.

26. Allen VG, Mitterni L, Seah C, et al. *Neisseria gonorrhoeae* treatment failure and susceptibility to cefixime in Toronto, Canada. JAMA 2013;309(2): 163–70.

27. Ohnishi M, Golparian D, Shimuta K, et al. Is *Neisseria gonorrhoeae* initiating a future era of untreatable gonorrhea?: detailed characterization of the first strain with high-level resistance to ceftriaxone. Antimicrobial Agents Chemother 2011; 55(7):3538–45.

28. Unemo M, Golparian D, Hestner A. Ceftriaxone treatment failure of pharyngeal gonorrhoea verified by international recommendations, Sweden, July 2010. Euro Surveill 2011;16(6). pii: 19792.

29. Unemo M, Golparian D, Potocnik M, et al. Treatment failure of pharyngeal gonorrhoea with internationally recommended first-line ceftriaxone verified in Slovenia, September 2011. Euro Surveill 2012;17(25). pii: 20200.

30. Carnicer-Pont D, Smithson A, Fina-Homar E, et al. First cases of *Neisseria gonorrhoeae* resistant to ceftriaxone in Catalonia, Spain, May 2011. Enferm Infecc Microbiol Clin 2012;30(4):218–9.
31. Unemo M, Shafer WM. Antibiotic resistance in *Neisseria gonorrhoeae*: origin, evolution, and lessons learned for the future. Ann N Y Acad Sci 2011;1230:E19–28.
32. Lindberg R, Fredlund H, Nicholas R, et al. *Neisseria gonorrhoeae* isolates with reduced susceptibility to cefixime and ceftriaxone: association with genetic polymorphisms in penA, mtrR, porB1b, and ponA. Antimicrobial Agents Chemother 2007;51(6):2117–22.
33. Wiesner PJ, Tronca E, Bonin P, et al. Clinical spectrum of pharyngeal gonococcal infection. N Engl J Med 1973;288(4):181–5.
34. Bro-Jorgensen A, Jensen T. Gonococcal pharyngeal infections. Report of 110 cases. Br J Vener Dis 1973;49(6):491–9.
35. Tice AW Jr, Rodriguez VL. Pharyngeal gonorrhea. JAMA 1981;246(23):2717–9.
36. Kinghorn G. Pharyngeal gonorrhoea: a silent cause for concern. Sex Transm Infect 2010;86(6):413–4.
37. Marcus JL, Bernstein KT, Kohn RP, et al. Infections missed by urethral-only screening for chlamydia or gonorrhea detection among men who have sex with men. Sex Transm Dis 2011;38(10):922–4.
38. Kent CK, Chaw JK, Wong W, et al. Prevalence of rectal, urethral, and pharyngeal chlamydia and gonorrhea detected in 2 clinical settings among men who have sex with men: San Francisco, California, 2003. Clin Infect Dis 2005;41(1):67–74.
39. Workowski KA, Berman S. Sexually transmitted diseases treatment guidelines, 2010. MMWR Recomm Rep 2010;59(RR-12):1–110.
40. Sulaiman MZ, Bates CM, Bittiner JB, et al. Response of pharyngeal gonorrhoea to single dose penicillin treatment. Genitourin Med 1987;63(2):92–4.
41. Ahmed-Jushuf IH, Bradley MG, Rao PM. Oropharyngeal carriage of *Neisseria gonorrhoeae* and its response to treatment in patients with anogenital infection. Genitourin Med 1988;64(1):64–5.
42. Handsfield HH, Knapp JS, Diehr PK, et al. Correlation of auxotype and penicillin susceptibility of *Neisseria gonorrhoeae* with sexual preference and clinical manifestations of gonorrhea. Sex Transm Dis 1980;7(1):1–5.
43. Giannini CM, Kim HK, Mortensen J, et al. Culture of non-genital sites increases the detection of gonorrhea in women. J Pediatr Adolesc Gynecol 2010;23(4):246–52.
44. Kinghorn GR, Rashid S. Prevalence of rectal and pharyngeal infection in women with gonorrhoea in Sheffield. Br J Vener Dis 1979;55(6):408–10.
45. Raychaudhuri M, Birley HD. Audit of routine rectal swabs for gonorrhoea culture in women. Int J STD AIDS 2010;21(2):143–4.
46. Javanbakht M, Gorbach P, Stirland A, et al. Prevalence and correlates of rectal chlamydia and gonorrhea among female clients at sexually transmitted disease clinics. Sex Transm Dis 2012;39(12):917–22.
47. Schachter J, Moncada J, Liska S, et al. Nucleic acid amplification tests in the diagnosis of chlamydial and gonococcal infections of the oropharynx and rectum in men who have sex with men. Sex Transm Dis 2008;35(7):637–42.
48. Bachmann LH, Johnson RE, Cheng H, et al. Nucleic acid amplification tests for diagnosis of *Neisseria gonorrhoeae* and *Chlamydia trachomatis* rectal infections. J Clin Microbiol 2010;48(5):1827–32.
49. Bachmann LH, Johnson RE, Cheng H, et al. Nucleic acid amplification tests for diagnosis of *Neisseria gonorrhoeae* oropharyngeal infections. J Clin Microbiol 2009;47(4):902–7.

50. Pandori M, Barry PM, Wu A, et al. Mosaic penicillin-binding protein 2 in *Neisseria gonorrhoeae* isolates collected in 2008 in San Francisco, California. Antimicrobial Agents Chemother 2009;53(9):4032–4.

51. Schachter J, Chernesky MA, Willis DE, et al. Vaginal swabs are the specimens of choice when screening for *Chlamydia trachomatis* and *Neisseria gonorrhoeae*: results from a multicenter evaluation of the APTIMA assays for both infections. Sex Transm Dis 2005;32(12):725–8.

52. Shafer MA, Moncada J, Boyer CB, et al. Comparing first-void urine specimens, self-collected vaginal swabs, and endocervical specimens to detect *Chlamydia trachomatis* and *Neisseria gonorrhoeae* by a nucleic acid amplification test. J Clin Microbiol 2003;41(9):4395–9.

53. Graseck AS, Shih SL, Peipert JF. Home versus clinic-based specimen collection for *Chlamydia trachomatis* and *Neisseria gonorrhoeae*. Expert Rev Anti Infect Ther 2011;9(2):183–94.

54. Rotblatt H, Montoya JA, Plant A, et al. There's no place like home: first-year use of the "I know" home testing program for chlamydia and gonorrhea. Am J Public Health 2013;103(8):1376–80.

55. Graseck AS, Secura GM, Allsworth JE, et al. Home screening compared with clinic-based screening for sexually transmitted infections. Obstet Gynecol 2010;115(4):745–52.

56. Chernesky MA, Hook EW 3rd, Martin DH, et al. Women find it easy and prefer to collect their own vaginal swabs to diagnose *Chlamydia trachomatis* or *Neisseria gonorrhoeae* infections. Sex Transm Dis 2005;32(12):729–33.

57. Wiesenfeld HC, Lowry DL, Heine RP, et al. Self-collection of vaginal swabs for the detection of Chlamydia, gonorrhea, and trichomoniasis: opportunity to encourage sexually transmitted disease testing among adolescents. Sex Transm Dis 2001;28(6):321–5.

58. Freeman AH, Bernstein KT, Kohn RP, et al. Evaluation of self-collected versus clinician-collected swabs for the detection of *Chlamydia trachomatis* and *Neisseria gonorrhoeae* pharyngeal infection among men who have sex with men. Sex Transm Dis 2011;38(11):1036–9.

59. Alexander S, Ison C, Parry J, et al. Self-taken pharyngeal and rectal swabs are appropriate for the detection of *Chlamydia trachomatis* and *Neisseria gonorrhoeae* in asymptomatic men who have sex with men. Sex Transm Infect 2008;84(6):488–92.

60. Sexton ME, Baker JJ, Nakagawa K, et al. How reliable is self-testing for gonorrhea and chlamydia among men who have sex with men? J Fam Pract 2013;62(2):70–8.

61. Wayal S, Llewellyn C, Smith H, et al. Home sampling kits for sexually transmitted infections: preferences and concerns of men who have sex with men. Cult Health Sex 2011;13(3):343–53.

62. Moran JS. Treating uncomplicated *Neisseria gonorrhoeae* infections: is the anatomic site of infection important? Sex Transm Dis 1995;22(1):39–47.

63. Moran JS, Levine WC. Drugs of choice for the treatment of uncomplicated gonococcal infections. Clin Infect Dis 1995;20(Suppl 1):S47–65.

64. Weinstock H, Workowski KA. Pharyngeal gonorrhea: an important reservoir of infection? Clin Infect Dis 2009;49(12):1798–800.

65. Whiley DM, Goire N, Lahra MM, et al. The ticking time bomb: escalating antibiotic resistance in *Neisseria gonorrhoeae* is a public health disaster in waiting. J Antimicrob Chemother 2012;67(9):2059–61.

66. Barbee LA, Kerani RP, Dombrowski JC, et al. A retrospective comparative study of two-drug oral and intramuscular cephalosporin treatment regimens for pharyngeal gonorrhea. Clin Infect Dis 2013;56(11):1539–45.

67. Sathia L, Ellis B, Phillip S, et al. Pharyngeal gonorrhoea—is dual therapy the way forward? Int J STD AIDS 2007;18(9):647–8.
68. Bignell C, Fitzgerald M. UK national guideline for the management of gonorrhoea in adults, 2011. Int J STD AIDS 2011;22(10):541–7.
69. Public Health Agency of Canada. Important notice on gonococcal infection. 2011. Available at: http://www.phac-aspc.gc.ca/std-mts/sti-its/alert/2011/alert-gono-eng.php. Accessed February 4, 2013.
70. Workowski K. Treatment in an era of dwindling treatment options. Oral presentation at the CDC National STD Prevention Conference 2012. Minneapolis, March 12–15, 2012.
71. Roblin PM, Kohlhoff SA, Parker C, et al. In vitro activity of CEM-101, a new fluoroketolide antibiotic, against *Chlamydia trachomatis* and *Chlamydia* (*Chlamydophila*) *pneumoniae*. Antimicrobial Agents Chemother 2010;54(3):1358–9.
72. Unemo M, Golparian D, Limnios A, et al. In vitro activity of ertapenem versus ceftriaxone against *Neisseria gonorrhoeae* isolates with highly diverse ceftriaxone MIC values and effects of ceftriaxone resistance determinants: ertapenem for treatment of gonorrhea? Antimicrobial Agents Chemother 2012;56(7):3603–9.
73. Brown LB, Krysiak R, Kamanga G, et al. *Neisseria gonorrhoeae* antimicrobial susceptibility in Lilongwe, Malawi, 2007. Sex Transm Dis 2010;37(3):169–72.
74. Dowell D, Kirkcaldy RD. Effectiveness of gentamicin for gonorrhoea treatment: systematic review and meta-analysis. Sex Transm Infect 2012;88(8):589–94.
75. Kircaldy R. Treatment of gonorrhea in an era of emerging cephalosporin resistance. STI & AIDS World Congress. Vienna, Austria, July 16, 2013.
76. Peterman TA, Tian LH, Metcalf CA, et al. High incidence of new sexually transmitted infections in the year following a sexually transmitted infection: a case for rescreening. Ann Intern Med 2006;145(8):564–72.
77. CDC. Cephalosporin-resistant *Neisseria gonorrhoeae* public health response plan. Atlanta (GA): Centers for Disease Control and Prevention; 2012.
78. Golden MR, Whittington WL, Handsfield HH, et al. Effect of expedited treatment of sex partners on recurrent or persistent gonorrhea or chlamydial infection. N Engl J Med 2005;352(7):676–85.
79. Zhu W, Chen CJ, Thomas CE, et al. Vaccines for gonorrhea: can we rise to the challenge? Front Microbiol 2011;2:124.

Screening and Management of Genital Chlamydial Infections

Devika Singh, MD, MPH[a],*, Jeanne M. Marrazzo, MD, MPH[b]

KEYWORDS

- Chlamydia • Screening • Chlamydial genital infection • Sexually transmitted disease

KEY POINTS

- Chlamydial genital infection is common and asymptomatic in most cases.
- National screening efforts developed to educate practitioners, expand screening, and link testing to local health laboratories are falling short of meeting the needs of populations at great risk of disease, including young racial/ethnic minority women and sexual minorities.
- The development and availability of newer diagnostics will likely make chlamydia testing more efficient and widely available for patients and providers.
- Practitioners are reminded to have a low threshold to offer testing and presumptive treatment to patients that are deemed at high risk of disease, particularly those who are challenging to engage in care.

INTRODUCTION

Chlamydia trachomatis is the most commonly reported notifiable disease in the United States and represents the largest proportion of sexually transmitted diseases (STDs) reported to the Centers for Disease Control and Prevention (CDC) since 1994.[1] Untreated chlamydial disease in women can ascend into the upper reproductive tract and place women at increased risk of human immunodeficiency virus (HIV) infection, ectopic pregnancy, infertility, and chronic pelvic pain. Despite its predisposition to cause severe disease and serious sequelae, particularly in young women, most individuals infected with chlamydia are asymptomatic. This fact has an obvious health impact and has prompted biomedical advances in testing and directed public health attention toward screening over the past few decades.

This article highlights the clinical manifestations, screening, and management of genital chlamydial infection in adults.

No commercial disclosures.
[a] Department of Global Health, Seattle STD/HIV Prevention Training Center (PTC), University of Washington, Box 359927, 325 Ninth Avenue, Seattle, WA 98104, USA; [b] Medicine/Division of Allergy and Infectious Diseases, Seattle STD/HIV Prevention Training Center (PTC), Harborview Medical Center, Box 359927, 325 Ninth Avenue, Seattle, WA 98104, USA
* Corresponding author.
E-mail address: dsingh@u.washington.edu

Infect Dis Clin N Am 27 (2013) 739–753
http://dx.doi.org/10.1016/j.idc.2013.08.006
0891-5520/13/$ – see front matter © 2013 Elsevier Inc. All rights reserved.

CLINICAL MANIFESTATIONS IN WOMEN

The most common genital clinical syndromes in women associated with *C trachomatis* include cervicitis, urethritis, pelvic inflammatory disease, and proctitis.

CERVICITIS

Most chlamydial infections involve the cervix.[2] To recognize the signs of cervical inflammation, one must understand the histologic changes that normally occur in the cervix during the reproductive period and menstrual cycle. The normal cervix of a young woman consists of 2 major kinds of epithelia: squamous and columnar.

Squamous epithelium covers most of the cervix and is contiguous with the vaginal epithelium. It is flat, pink, and opaque, rather like the lining of the mouth. Columnar epithelium, redder in appearance, may be confined to the endocervical canal or may be found surrounding the cervical os, where it is often referred to as *ectopy*. Ectopy is commonly seen in young women (typically women <25 years old) and in women using oral contraceptives. Ectopy is thought to increase the risk of infection through exposing columnar epithelium to an infectious pathogen, such as *C trachomatis*.

Factors that define the syndrome of cervicitis include endocervical discharge that is mucopurulent, increased in amount, and exhibits an increased number of polymorphonuclear leukocytes (PMNs) (>30 PMNs/1000× field) on endocervical gram stain. Easily induced endocervical bleeding (defined as sustained bleeding on gentle passage of a nonabrasive swab, such as cotton or polyester) and the presence of edematous ectopy are also cardinal signs.

However, most endocervical chlamydial infections—at least 80% to 85%—occur without any signs or symptoms of disease. This fact has prompted recommendations for routine annual screening among sexually active women younger than 26 years.[3] Both the CDC and U.S. Preventive Services Task Force (USPSTF) also endorse screening of older women with risk factors (eg, those who have a new sex partner or multiple sex partners). In June 2007, the USPSTF made the decision to alter the age groups used to demonstrate disease incidence (ie, from persons aged ≤25 years to those aged ≤24 years) based on their review of the data.[4]

URETHRITIS

Approximately 25% of women with chlamydial cervicitis have concomitant urethritis, often with associated dysuria-pyuria. Although some women may complain of symptoms typical of cystitis, most are asymptomatic. Findings on urinalysis generally include some degree of pyuria without bacteria or organisms. Bacterial cultures are usually unrevealing. Other causes to consider in the setting of pyuria without bacteriuria include infection with *N gonorrhoeae*, herpes simplex virus (HSV), or lower-colony-count urinary tract infections.

PELVIC INFLAMMATORY DISEASE

Pelvic inflammatory disease (PID) is a term used to describe upper genital tract infections that frequently involve the endometrium (endometritis), fallopian tubes (salpingitis or tubo-ovarian abscess), and pelvic peritoneum (peritonitis). These infections result from ascending spread of lower genital tract infection.

Infection of the upper genital tract is estimated to occur in roughly one-fourth of women who do undergo treatment of their chlamydial cervical infection.[5] Upper tract infection caused by chlamydia can be clinically silent much of the time. Moreover, PID from chlamydia is associated with higher rates of clinical sequelae, including infertility, ectopic pregnancy, and chronic pelvic pain. The clinical manifestations, diagnosis, and treatment of PID are discussed separately.

CLINICAL MANIFESTATIONS IN MEN

The clinical manifestations of genital chlamydia infection in men include urethritis, epididymitis, prostatitis, and proctitis.

URETHRITIS

Urethritis is the most frequent STD syndrome in men. It is characterized by urethral inflammation and has traditionally been classified as gonococcal or nongonococcal urethritis (NGU). *C trachomatis* is the causative agent in 15% to 40% of cases. Other potential pathogens in urethritis include *N gonorrhoeae, Mycoplasma genitalium* (seems to account for 15%–25% of NGU cases in the United States), *Trichomonas vaginalis*, HSV, and adenovirus. Support for other *Mycoplasma* and *Ureaplasma* species being causative pathogens in urethritis remains inconsistent. Most patients with urethritis from genital herpes infection will have obvious herpetic penile lesions, and many with urethritis from *T vaginalis* will have sex partners that also have this infection.

Standard recommendations have been to treat NGU with 1 g of azithromycin, not only because historically there has been little concern for reduced efficacy but also because of the known advantage of greater adherence and directly observed improvement associated with a single-dose regimen. More recently, however, some study results have challenged the most optimal treatment for urethritis in men. One multicenter randomized controlled trial comparing azithromycin or doxycycline with or without tinidazole (to eradicate possible trichomoniasis infection) showed a treatment efficacy of only 77% among the 53 men who received azithromycin, compared with 95% of the 58 patients who received doxycycline (*P* = .011).[6] Another recently published study collected more than 4 years' worth of data in a parallel-group superiority design comparing the treatment of NGU with either azithromycin or doxycycline among men attending an STD clinic in Seattle.[7] In modified intent-to-treat analyses, 172 of 216 (80%; 95% confidence interval [CI], 74%–85%) of men receiving azithromycin and 157 of 206 (76%; 95% CI, 70%–82%) of men receiving doxycycline experienced clinical cure (*P* = .40), exhibiting low clinical cure rates and no difference between the regimens.

EPIDIDYMITIS

The classic presentation of acute epididymitis includes unilateral, severe testicular pain and tenderness, and swelling of the epididymis felt on palpation. Objective findings include

- Gram stain of urethral secretions demonstrating 5 or more white blood cells (WBCs) per oil immersion field. Gram stain is the preferred rapid diagnostic test for evaluating urethritis because it is highly sensitive and specific for documenting both urethritis and the presence or absence of gonococcal infection. Gonococcal infection is established by documenting the presence of WBCs containing intracellular gram-negative diplococci on urethral Gram stain.
- Positive leukocyte esterase test on first-void urine, or microscopic examination of first-void urine sediment demonstrating 10 or more WBCs per high-power field.

Although radionuclide scanning of the scrotum can confirm the clinical finding of epididymitis with the greatest accuracy, it is neither commonly available nor cost-efficient for diagnosis. Ultrasonography, similarly, is highly sensitive for diagnosing acute epididymitis and may be useful to rule out testicular torsion in the setting of acute severe unilateral pain.

Evaluation and empiric coverage of both chlamydia and gonorrhea is appropriate, because these are the most frequently recovered pathogens in sexually acquired epididymitis.

PROSTATITIS

Although more research on this topic is warranted, C trachomatis has been reported in some cases of chronic prostatitis. A few studies involving in situ hybridization and detection of chlamydia antigen show recovery of chlamydia more frequently in urine and prostatic secretions compared with controls.[8–10] A 4-year study of chlamydial infection among U.S. Air Force personnel showed a significant risk for development of prostatitis among those who tested positive for chlamydia.[11]

PROCTITIS/PROCTOCOLITIS

The term proctitis refers to inflammation of the rectal mucosa (ie, the distal 10–12 cm). Classically, symptoms are similar to those associated with urinary tract infection and include increased urinary frequency, urgency, and dysuria. Practitioners ought to consider chlamydial proctitis in women and men who acknowledge receptive anal intercourse. Patients may also complain of constipation, tenesmus, rectal discomfort or pain, passage of bloody stools, and a mucopurulent rectal discharge, which is occasionally misinterpreted by the patient as diarrhea. Findings on rectal examination generally reveal exquisite tenderness. Anoscopy or sigmoidoscopy may reveal the presence of mucus to diffuse inflammation of the mucosa with friability or discrete ulcerations. If the mucosa is abnormal, extending to 12 cm above the anus, then proctocolitis is present. A rectal biopsy can provide histologic confirmation of proctitis and may reveal nonspecific inflammation or changes highly suggestive of certain infections, such as gonorrhea, lymphogranuloma venereum (LGV), HSV, or syphilis.

Chlamydia proctitis and other sexually transmitted gastrointestinal syndromes caused by syphilis, gonorrhea, HSV, and human papillomavirus became very common in the 1970s and early 1980s among men who have sex with men (MSM). Their incidence decreased over the next couple of decades, probably because of increased safer sex practices. However, in the late 1990s, rectal bacterial STDs increased markedly among MSM in many cities in the United States and Europe. Transmission of these pathogens is facilitated by exposure to multiple sexual partners, specific sexual practices (especially anal intercourse and anilingus), and the ability of small inocula of these agents to cause infection.

Diagnostic methods for proctitis include gram-stained smear of the rectal mucosa obtained during anoscopy (≥ 1 PMN/$1000\times$ oil immersion field) and rectal cultures for gonorrhea, chlamydia, and HSV. Nucleic acid amplification tests (NAAT) are not currently approved by the U.S. Food and Drug Administration (FDA) for use on nongenital specimens, but many laboratories have established performance specifications (Clinical Laboratory Improvement Amendments [CLIA] standards) for rectal NAATs.

LGV

The L1, L2, and L3 serovars of *C trachomatis* cause the disease known as LGV. These serovars differ from those (D–K) that cause the more common sexually transmitted chlamydial infections (urethritis and cervicitis). Because the clinical course of LGV proctitis can vary from indolent to severe, manifesting with bloody and purulent rectal discharge and tenesmus, the condition might not be suspected early during the course of illness, and diagnosis can be delayed. Because the rectal symptoms of LGV can be severe, including perirectal abscesses, referral to a gastroenterologist for colonoscopy or sigmoidoscopy to rule out inflammatory bowel disease has some-times preceded identification of the correct diagnosis.

Pharyngeal Infection

The common use of newer diagnostic tests that target both *N gonorrhoeae* and *C trachomatis* has resulted in frequent "reflex" performance of chlamydia testing on pharyngeal swab specimens intended for gonorrhea testing. Thus, the clinician is faced with a positive test result from an anatomic niche that is not known to be a major reservoir for chlamydial infection, or to experience adverse consequences from it. Some investigators argue that detection of the pathogen at this site does not even really represent an infection, per se, because no human or animal models for patho-genesis or infectivity exist at this site. Detection of the organism at this site may rep-resent recent sexual exposure. For this reason, and because more research must be performed, the authors recommend treatment with a standard regimen for uncompli-cated chlamydial infection if a pharyngeal test results are positive. Sex partners should be managed as for a genital infection, discussed later.

DIAGNOSIS

Several methods are available for diagnosing chlamydia, including NAAT, antigen detection, unamplified genetic probes, and culture. NAAT may be used for urine, vaginal swabs, endocervical swabs, and, although not formally cleared by the FDA, rectal samples. Laboratories can achieve CLIA compliance to satisfy regulations for rectal and oropharyngeal testing (available at: http://www.aphl.org/aphlprograms/infectious/std/Documents/CTGCLabGuidelinesMeetingReport.pdf).

Noninvasive testing involving urine collection and self-collected vaginal discharge is becoming increasingly standard in a variety of settings, with considerable support for its enhanced sensitivity to both urine and endocervical swabs using NAAT.[12] More-over, self-collected rectal swabs have been shown to be highly acceptable to both women and MSM.[13,14]

NAAT

These assays include polymerase chain reaction (PCR) amplification of chlamydia DNA or RNA, transcription-mediated amplification (TMA), and strand displacement assay (SDA). NAATs have largely replaced other historic methods of diagnosis and are considered the gold standard. Considerable evidence shows the high sensitivity and specificity of NAAT for chlamydia. One large review of pooled data from 29 studies revealed that the sensitivity and specificity of urine testing compared with invasive testing (urethral sampling):

- PCR assays (14 studies): the pooled sensitivity and specificity were 83.0% and 99.5% for urine samples and 86.0% and 99.6% for cervical samples.

- TMA assay (4 studies): the pooled sensitivity and specificity were 93% and 99% for urine samples and 97% and 99% for cervical samples.
- SDA assay (2 studies): the pooled sensitivity and specificity were 80% and 99% for urine samples and 94% and 98% for cervical samples.

Other testing modalities are used far less frequently, primarily because of their reliance on invasive methods (antigen detection and genetic probes require a swab from the cervix or urethra) and, more importantly, their relative insensitivity. Recent interest has been shown in rapid testing given the desire for same-day results and also the expense and lack of availability of NAAT in resource-limited settings. Although not available in the United States, the Chlamydia Rapid Test, used in first-void urine in men, exhibited moderate sensitivity (82.6%), specificity (98.5%), and positive (84.1%) and negative predictive (98.3%) values compared with PCR.[15]

Definitive diagnosis of LGV proctitis is challenging. Although direct testing on rectal mucosal specimens for *C trachomatis* is indicated, the FDA has approved only cell culture for this purpose. However, cell culture is not widely available, is expensive, and is technically difficult to interpret. As stated earlier, NAAT is not FDA-approved for rectal specimens, but may be used in laboratories that meet validation specifications. Information about the process to obtain this validation can be found at www.cdc.gov/std/ *C trachomatis* serology (complement fixation titers>1:64) can support the diagnosis of LGV in an appropriate clinical context but is performed infrequently, is not standardized, and requires a high level of expertise to interpret. It may also not diagnose rectal infections in men as well as it does upper genital tract infection in women.

SCREENING

Apparent increases in rates of chlamydia in the developed world reflect several factors, including a likely increase in disease burden, in combination with expanded national screening efforts, enhanced use of highly sensitive diagnostic tests, and overall improvements in case reporting by providers, laboratories, and public health programs. Despite clear national screening guidelines, challenges remain in achieving target screening levels at a population level.

The Healthcare Effectiveness Data and Information Set (HEDIS) assesses screening coverage for chlamydia among the young women who receive care through either commercial or Medicaid managed care organizations. Findings from an analysis of HEDIS data revealed that among sexually active women aged 16 to 24 years enrolled in commercial plans, screening increased from 23.1% in 2001 to 43.1% in 2010. Among the same age group of women covered by Medicaid, screening increased from 40.4% to 57.5%.[16] Although these estimates and those of the National Survey of Family Growth (NSFG) are considered fairly reliable measures of screening practices, more recent analyses suggests that these methods may actually underestimate screening coverage. In an analysis of data conducted at the University of Washington using estimates from the census, HEDIS, and NSFG, researchers suggest that health departments can extrapolate population-level screening more comprehensively using data drawn from tested samples in large laboratories.[17]

EPIDEMIOLOGY

The total rate of chlamydia for the United States in 2011 was 457.6 per 100,000 according to the CDC, representing an increase of 8.0% since 2010. The greatest burden of chlamydial infection is in young women, as evidenced by a prevalence of approximately 6.8% in sexually active women aged 14 to 19 years.[18]

Several populations capture particular national interest in the context of STD and HIV prevention, including young adults (particularly young women), racial and ethnic minorities, and sexual minorities. The highest burden of chlamydial disease is in young women and some racial/ethnic minority populations. Estimates are more uncertain for chlamydial PID because of the imprecise nature of the clinical diagnosis, and also probably because of underreporting. Per the CDC's National Data Discharge Survey data from 2010, hospitalizations from PID seemed to decline between the 1980s and 1990s, but stabilized between 2000 and 2007 (**Fig. 1**).

YOUNG WOMEN

According to the CDC, the overall rate of reported chlamydia in 2011 among women was more than and a half times the rate among men (658.9 cases per 100,000 among women and 256.9 cases per 100,000 among men). The highest rates of reported chlamydia in 2011 were among younger women, with 3722.5 cases per 100,000 women versus 1343.3 cases per 100,000 men ages 20 to 24 years, and 3416.5 cases per 100,000 women versus 689.7 cases per 100,000 men ages 15 to 19 years.

RACE/ETHNICITY

Populations based on race/ethnicity that seem to be impacted disproportionately by chlamydial disease include Blacks/African Americans and American Indians/Alaska Natives (AI/AN). Rates among Blacks was more than 7 times the rate among whites (1194.4 and 159.0 cases per 100,000, respectively). The rate among American Indians/Alaska natives was more than 4 times the rate among whites (648.3 cases per 100,000). An analysis using a dataset of more than 7300 patient visits for chlamydia testing in the Pacific Northwest during 1997 through 2004 revealed that chlamydia positivity increased upwards of 2.2 times that of the non-AI/AN population, with an increase in reported risk behaviors and younger age among those tested over the study period.[19] Moreover, consistent with racial disparities in gonorrhea and chlamydia, rates of PID are 2 to 3 times higher among Black women than among White women (**Fig. 2**).[20]

SEXUAL MINORITY POPULATIONS

According to the 2006–2008 NSFG, 13% of women and 5.2% of men aged 15 to 44 years reported same-sex behavior in their lifetime.[21] Women who have sex with women (WSW) represent diverse communities of women who may exclusively have

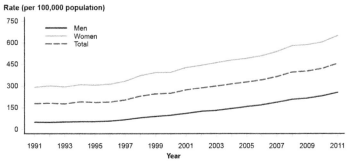

Fig. 1. Chlamydia rates by sex, United States, 1991–2011. (*Courtesy of* The Centers for Disease Control and Prevention. Available at: http://www.cdc.gov/std/stats11/figures/1.htm.)

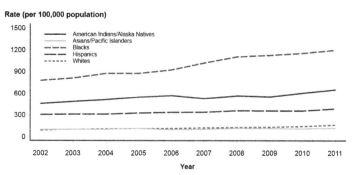

Fig. 2. Chlamydia rates by race/ethnicity, United States, 2002–2011. (*Courtesy of* The Centers for Disease Control and Prevention. Available at: http://www.cdc.gov/std/stats11/figures/6. htm.)

sex with women, or historically (or currently) engage in sexual partnerships with both men and women. Despite the fact that same-sex behavior is not infrequent among women in the United States, and despite the widespread prevalence of chlamydia, few data at the clinic, community, or population levels are available that describe its prevalence among these sexual minority communities.

Although incident HIV infection and several unsafe sexual practices declined from the 1980s into the 1990s, more recent data suggest that several STD are increasing among MSM, including chlamydia.[22,23] Several high-risk sexual behaviors among some subgroups of MSM seem to be associated with higher rates of STD, including decreased safer-sex precautions ("prevention fatigue"); illicit drug use, especially methamphetamine use; dynamic patterns within sexual networks (eg, meeting sex partners online) that promote more anonymous partnerships; and an evolving trend of seeking sexual partners of the same serostatus ("serosorting").

WSW

Women aged 15 to 24 years attending family planning clinics in the U.S. Pacific Northwest during 1997 through 2005 and who reported same-sex behavior had higher positivity of *C trachomatis* than those who reported exclusively heterosexual behavior.[24] Factors associated with chlamydial infection detection among WSW in this study included the use of NAATs for diagnosis, testing at a non–routine visit, report of genitourinary symptoms, and report of a sex partner with chlamydial infection. Over the study period, WSW who reported sexual behavioral risks also had the highest chlamydia positivity compared with those who had sex exclusively with men or those who had sex with men and women who reported similar risks. A greater proportion of women who had sex with men and women reported sexual behavioral risks compared with both heterosexual women and those who had sex only with women; despite this, chlamydia positivity was not highest in this group. Researchers also noted a high chlamydia positivity among American Indian/Alaska Native women who reported sex with women, a finding that is consistent with racial/ethnic disparities described previously from the Region × Infertility Prevention Project (IPP) data.[19] The finding of higher chlamydia positivity among WSW relative to women reporting sex exclusively with men was unexpected. Possible explanations for this observation relate to differences in these groups' use of reproductive health care services (including chlamydia screening), biologic susceptibility to lower genital tract infection, infrequent use of barrier methods to prevent STD transmission with female partners, trends toward higher-risk behaviors, and different characteristics of their respective sexual networks.

Taken together, these data emphasize that WSW should undergo routine age-based annual screening for *C trachomatis* as recommended by current guidelines.

MSM

Standard guidelines from the CDC urge clinicians to sensitively explore STD risk behaviors and review patient-centered prevention methods among all MSM, including those with HIV infection.[3] Beyond this, knowing the local epidemiology for a particular STD, including chlamydia, is helpful in understanding risk profiles for individual patients within broader sexual networks. Eliciting a comprehensive sexual history includes inquiring about number and sex of partners, HIV status of partners, use of safer-sex methods (eg, condoms, female condoms, dental dams), types of sexual activity (eg, oral sex, anal sex), role in sexual partnerships (eg, insertive vs receptive), any associated drug use (including alcohol), and contexts of sexual encounters (eg, bath houses, Internet). Clinicians should routinely ask about common STD-associated symptoms, including urethral discharge, dysuria, anal pain or discharge, genital or anal ulcers, swollen or painful lymph nodes, fevers, sweats, and rash.

To reduce the risk of acquisition and transmission of HIV, the CDC specifies that STD screening should include annual urethral/urine screening for both gonorrhea and chlamydia among sexually active MSM, pharyngeal gonorrhea cultures for MSM with oral-genital exposure, and rectal chlamydia and gonorrhea cultures for MSM who engage in receptive anal sex.[3] Despite the CDC's intentions and public health efforts to adhere to these guidelines, historically few STD clinics and gay men's health centers have offered rectal chlamydial screening for asymptomatic MSM.[25] One study that evaluated the prevalence of chlamydial and gonorrhea infections among MSM in San Francisco, California[23] applied previously validated NAATs to specimens obtained from the pharynx, rectum, and urethra. These investigators found that 85% of rectal gonorrhea and chlamydia occurred in asymptomatic men. Moreover, 53% of chlamydial infections occurred at nonurethral sites and would have been missed if only urethral/urine screening was performed. Finally, more than 70% of chlamydial infections would have been missed and left untreated if only gonorrhea testing occurred. Another study showed the prevalence of rectal chlamydial infection to be 9% by culture and 23% by NAAT among MSM reporting receptive anal intercourse in an urban STD clinic in a Midwestern US city. Additionally, a significant association was seen between HIV status and rectal chlamydia.[26]

Researchers from the CDC and the San Francisco Department of Public Health examined 2 different statistical models and found that rectal screening of chlamydia and gonorrhea is a potentially cost-effective intervention to prevent HIV infection among high-risk MSM who practice anal sex.[27] Moreover, in a study conducted in an urban STD clinic in Melbourne, Australia, outreach in the form of automatic, computer-generated reminders was associated with increased detection of bacterial sexually transmitted infections (STIs), including both urethral and rectal chlamydia, among MSM.[28] Given that both gonorrhea and chlamydia increase the risk of HIV acquisition and transmission, settings that conduct STI testing should optimize screening and treatment of asymptomatic MSM at all relevant anatomic sites, ideally with the use of NAATs.

LGV

LGV has been steadily gaining clinical and public health attention over the past several years. In 2004, public health officials in the Netherlands reported a case of a young man with ulcerative proctitis caused by a rare strain of C trachomatis.[29,30] The current exact number of cases of LGV in the United States is unknown, owing largely to the challenges in its diagnostics. Historically, LGV has been recognized as an STD among travelers returning from the Caribbean or other tropical areas, but those cases generally run a benign course with finding of a mild genital ulcer followed by development of inguinal lymphadenopathy (buboes).

Large-scale outbreaks of LGV proctitis have been documented in New York City[31] and the United Kingdom,[32] concentrated in communities of MSM who are active in anal sex. Notable public health concern exists regarding diagnoses of other concomitant STI in these contexts. In an outbreak of LGV described in the United Kingdom among 282 MSM, most (96%) had proctitis, with either severe or systemic symptoms, and a high level of coinfection was documented with HIV (76%), hepatitis C (19%), and other STDs (39%).[32] Persons diagnosed with LGV should undergo testing for HIV and other STDs. MSM diagnosed with LGV should also undergo testing for hepatitis B and C.

Although lower gastrointestinal/rectal manifestations may some bring persons to clinical attention, high rates of asymptomatic rectal chlamydia infection also occur among communities of MSM.[33] This fact indicates the need for rigorous and targeted screening programs, given that outreach and diagnosis of LGV among high risk communities in combination with effective treatment will help address broader screening goals including STD prevention.

TREATMENT

Treatment of patients diagnosed with chlamydia effectively prevents transmission of the disease. Moreover, treatment of all sex partners (within the past 60 days of diagnosis) helps prevent reinfection and spread to other partners. Finally, treatment of pregnant women prevents transmission of C trachomatis to infants during birth. Newer testing technologies are emerging to allow for early treatment for persons testing positive for infection. Delays in treatment may lead to preventable complications. Syndromes consistent with a chlamydial origin, including cervicitis, urethritis, and epididymitis, should be treated with an antibiotic regimen that includes activity against chlamydia. This management is especially important given chlamydia's relatively high prevalence and potential for causing complications, such as PID and other adverse sequelae.

The efficacy of recommended regimens for treating chlamydial infection is high. A meta-analysis of a dozen randomized clinical trials evaluating azithromycin versus doxycycline for the treatment of genital chlamydial infection showed microbial cure rates of 97% and 98%, respectively.[34]

Patients who experience persistent symptoms after therapy with either azithromycin or doxycycline and assert full adherence are not likely experiencing treatment failure. A study that followed a cohort of adolescent women performed NAAT testing and ompA genotyping to evaluate for rates of chlamydia reinfection or persistent infection. A total of 478 chlamydial infections were detected in 210 participants, with 176 who remained uninfected throughout the duration of the study. Most (84.2%) infections were likely reinfections, whereas 13.7% were documented as possible or probable treatment failures, and a minority (2.2%) was categorized as chlamydial infections despite appropriate recommended treatment.[35]

Abundant data support the safety and efficacy of azithromycin in pregnant women.[36,37] Test-of-cure ought to occur (using NAAT, if available) 3 weeks after completion of therapy for all pregnant women diagnosed with chlamydia. Also, per the United States Preventive Services Task Force (USPSTF), other populations of women deemed at increased risk for chlamydia (eg, those aged <25 years, those who have a new or

---

Box 1
Empiric treatment for gonorrhea and chlamydia while awaiting diagnostic test results

- Ceftriaxone, 250 mg intramuscularly in a single dose

    PLUS EITHER

- Azithromycin, 1.0 g orally in a single dose

    OR

- Doxycycline, 100 mg orally twice daily for 7 days

Targeted *C trachomatis* treatment

  Recommended regimen

- Azithromycin, 1.0 g orally in a single dose

      OR

- Doxycycline, 100 mg orally twice daily for 7 days

  Alternative regimens

- Erythromycin, 500 mg orally 4 times daily for 7 days
- Erythromycin ethylsuccinate, 800 mg orally 4 times daily for 7 days
- Levofloxacin, 500 mg orally every day for 7 days
- Ofloxacin, 300 mg orally twice daily for 7 days

Recommended regimens in pregnancy

  Azithromycin, 1.0 g orally in a single dose

    OR

  Amoxicillin, 500 mg orally 3 times daily for 7 days

Alternative regimens

  Erythromycin base, 500 mg orally 4 times daily for 7 days

    OR

  Erythromycin base, 250 mg orally 4 times daily for 14 days

    OR

  Erythromycin ethylsuccinate, 800 mg orally 4 times daily for 7 days

    OR

  Erythromycin ethylsuccinate, 400 mg orally 4 times daily for 14 days

Proctitis

  Chlamydial infection (LGV strains)

- Doxycycline, 100 mg twice daily for 3 weeks

  Chlamydial infection (non-LGV strains)

- Doxycycline, 100 mg twice daily for 7 to 10 days

  Pregnancy/lactation

- Erythromycin base, 500 mg orally 4 times daily for 21 days

---

multiple sex partners) should undergo retesting during the third trimester to prevent maternal postnatal complications. Finally, given that doxycycline is FDA pregnancy category D, historic support exists for erythromycin treatment in both pregnant and lactating women diagnosed with LGV.[38]

Current clinical guidance from the CDC for clinicians, particularly those who care for HIV-infected MSM, emphasizes the need to be alert for rectal signs and symptoms suggestive of proctitis. Clinicians who suspect a case of LGV proctitis should seek expert advice from local public health authorities and infectious disease specialists on how to diagnose the condition effectively. Often, given the lack of available local expertise, this is not possible. In these cases, an empiric course of therapy is warranted (**Box 1**). LGV responds well to doxycycline, but the drug must be given for 3 weeks (100 mg orally twice daily)—a longer course than required for non-LGV chlamydial infection—to be effective.

FOLLOW-UP

Posttreatment test-of-cure (repeat testing 3–4 weeks after completion of therapy) is not routinely performed when recommended regimens (azithromycin or doxycycline) are used for treatment of chlamydia. Instead, practitioners are encouraged to pursue test-of-cure in the following scenarios:

- In pregnant patients
- When adherence to therapy is in question
- When symptoms persist despite therapy
- When reinfection is suspected

Use of NAAT may yield false-positive results because of the ongoing presence of nonviable organisms if used within less than 3 weeks from completion of therapy, challenging its validity in this context. For this reason, test-of-cure should not be performed using NAAT until 3 weeks after completion of therapy.

The CDC recommends that persons diagnosed with chlamydia undergo retesting approximately 3 months after treatment, despite sex partner treatment status. If meeting this time frame presents a challenge, retesting should occur whenever the patient next presents for medical care in the subsequent 12 months after initial treatment.

All sexual contacts within the past 60 days of persons with *C trachomatis* infection should treated with doxycycline, 100 mg orally twice daily for 7 days, or azithromycin, 1.0 g orally once. Patient-delivered partner therapy (PDPT) can be a highly effective means to ensure treatment of heterosexual partners who may be less likely to present for care. Currently, PDPT is not routinely recommended for MSM because of a high risk for coexisting infections, especially undiagnosed HIV infection, in their partners.

Patients undergoing treatment for LGV should be followed clinically until signs and symptoms have resolved. Sexual contacts of those undergoing treatment for LGV within the past 60 days ought to undergo testing for urethral (or cervical) chlamydial infection and treated (azithromycin, 1 g orally in a single dose, or doxycycline, 100 mg orally twice daily for 7 days).

SUMMARY

Chlamydial genital infection is common and asymptomatic in most cases. National screening efforts developed to educate practitioners, expand screening, and link testing to local health laboratories are not meeting the needs of populations at great risk of disease, including young racial/ethnic minority women and sexual minorities. The development and availability of newer diagnostics will likely make chlamydia testing more efficient and widely available for patients and providers. Practitioners are reminded to have a low threshold to offer testing and presumptive treatment to patients who are deemed at high risk of disease, particularly those who are challenging to engage in care.

REFERENCES

1. Centers for Disease Control and Prevention. Sexually Transmitted Disease Surveillance, 2010. Atlanta (GA): CDC; Department of Health and Human Services; 2011.
2. WE S. Chlamydia trachomatis infections of the adult. In: Holmes KK, Sparling PF, Stamm WE, et al, editors. Sexually transmitted diseases. 4th edition. New York: McGraw-Hill; 2008. p. 575–95.
3. Workowski KA, Berman S, Centers for Disease Control and Prevention (CDC). Sexually transmitted diseases treatment guidelines, 2010. MMWR Recomm Rep 2010;59(RR-12):1–110.
4. Meyers DS, et al. Screening for chlamydial infection: an evidence update for the U.S. Preventive Services Task Force. Ann Intern Med 2007;147(2):135–42.
5. Wiesenfeld HC, et al. Lower genital tract infection and endometritis: insight into subclinical pelvic inflammatory disease. Obstet Gynecol 2002;100(3):456–63.
6. Schwebke JR, et al. Re-evaluating the treatment of nongonococcal urethritis: emphasizing emerging pathogens–a randomized clinical trial. Clin Infect Dis 2011;52(2):163–70.
7. Manhart LE, et al. Standard treatment regimens for nongonococcal urethritis have similar but declining cure rates: a randomized controlled trial. Clin Infect Dis 2013;56(7):934–42.
8. Mutlu N, et al. The role of Chlamydia trachomatis in patients with non-bacterial prostatitis. Int J Clin Pract 1998;52(8):540–1.
9. Ostaszewska I. Chlamydia trachomatis as a probable cause of prostatitis. Int J STD AIDS 2000;11(7):482–3.
10. Gumus B, et al. Evaluation of non-invasive clinical samples in chronic chlamydial prostatitis by using in situ hybridization. Scand J Urol Nephrol 1997;31(5):449–51.
11. Trei JS, Canas LC, Gould PL. Reproductive tract complications associated with Chlamydia trachomatis infection in US Air Force males within 4 years of testing. Sex Transm Dis 2008;35(9):827–33.
12. Hobbs MM, et al. From the NIH: proceedings of a workshop on the importance of self-obtained vaginal specimens for detection of sexually transmitted infections. Sex Transm Dis 2008;35(1):8–13.
13. van der Helm JJ, et al. High performance and acceptability of self-collected rectal swabs for diagnosis of Chlamydia trachomatis and Neisseria gonorrhoeae in men who have sex with men and women. Sex Transm Dis 2009; 36(8):493–7.
14. Freeman AH, et al. Evaluation of self-collected versus clinician-collected swabs for the detection of Chlamydia trachomatis and Neisseria gonorrhoeae pharyngeal infection among men who have sex with men. Sex Transm Dis 2011; 38(11):1036–9.
15. Nadala EC, et al. Performance evaluation of a new rapid urine test for chlamydia in men: prospective cohort study. BMJ 2009;339:b2655.
16. National Committee for Quality Assurance. HEDIS 2013: technical specifications. Washington, DC: National Committee for Quality Assurance; 2012. p. 90–3.
17. Broad JM, et al. Chlamydia screening coverage estimates derived using healthcare effectiveness data and information system procedures and indirect estimation vary substantially. Sex Transm Dis 2013;40(4):292–7.
18. Centers for Disease Control and Prevention (CDC). CDC Grand Rounds: Chlamydia prevention: challenges and strategies for reducing disease burden and sequelae. MMWR Morb Mortal Wkly Rep 2011;60(12):370–3.

19. Gorgos L, Fine D, Marrazzo J. Chlamydia positivity in American Indian/Alaska Native women screened in family planning clinics, 1997–2004. Sex Transm Dis 2008;35(8):753–7.
20. Sutton MY, et al. Trends in pelvic inflammatory disease hospital discharges and ambulatory visits, United States, 1985–2001. Sex Transm Dis 2005;32(12): 778–84.
21. Chandra A, et al. Sexual behavior, sexual attraction, and sexual identity in the United States: data from the 2006-2008 National Survey of Family Growth. Natl Health Stat Report 2011;(36):1–36.
22. Mayer KH, Klausner JD, Handsfield HH. Intersecting epidemics and educable moments: sexually transmitted disease risk assessment and screening in men who have sex with men. Sex Transm Dis 2001;28(8):464–7.
23. Kent CK, et al. Prevalence of rectal, urethral, and pharyngeal chlamydia and gonorrhea detected in 2 clinical settings among men who have sex with men: San Francisco, California, 2003. Clin Infect Dis 2005;41(1):67–74.
24. Singh D, Fine D, Marrazzo C. Chlamydia trachomatis infection among women reporting sex with women screened in family planning clinics in the Pacific Northwest, 1997–2005. Am J Public Health 2011;101:1284–90.
25. Battle TJ, et al. Evaluation of laboratory testing methods for Chlamydia trachomatis infection in the era of nucleic acid amplification. J Clin Microbiol 2001;39(8): 2924–7.
26. Turner AN, et al. HIV, rectal chlamydia, and rectal gonorrhea in men who have sex with men attending a sexually transmitted disease clinic in a Midwestern US City. Sex Transm Dis 2013;40(6):433–8.
27. Chesson HW BK, Gift TL, Marcus JL, et al. The cost-effectiveness of screening men who have sex with men for rectal chlamydial and gonococcal infection to prevent HIV infection. Sex Transm Dis 2013;40(5):366–71.
28. Zou H, et al. Automated, computer generated reminders and increased detection of gonorrhoea, Chlamydia and syphilis in men who have sex with men. PLoS One 2013;8(4):e61972.
29. Nieuwenhuis RF, et al. Resurgence of lymphogranuloma venereum in Western Europe: an outbreak of Chlamydia trachomatis serovar l2 proctitis in The Netherlands among men who have sex with men. Clin Infect Dis 2004;39(7): 996–1003.
30. Nieuwenhuis RF, et al. Unusual presentation of early lymphogranuloma venereum in an HIV-1 infected patient: effective treatment with 1 g azithromycin. Sex Transm Infect 2003;79(6):453–5.
31. Pathela P, Blank S, Schillinger JA. Lymphogranuloma venereum: old pathogen, new story. Curr Infect Dis Rep 2007;9(2):143–50.
32. Ward H, et al. Lymphogranuloma venereum in the United kingdom. Clin Infect Dis 2007;44(1):26–32.
33. Annan NT, et al. Rectal chlamydia–a reservoir of undiagnosed infection in men who have sex with men. Sex Transm Infect 2009;85(3):176–9.
34. Lau CY, Qureshi AK. Azithromycin versus doxycycline for genital chlamydial infections: a meta-analysis of randomized clinical trials. Sex Transm Dis 2002; 29(9):497–502.
35. Batteiger BE, et al. Repeated Chlamydia trachomatis genital infections in adolescent women. J Infect Dis 2010;201(1):42–51.
36. Jacobson GF, et al. A randomized controlled trial comparing amoxicillin and azithromycin for the treatment of Chlamydia trachomatis in pregnancy. Am J Obstet Gynecol 2001;184(7):1352–4 [discussion: 1354–6].

37. Rahangdale L, et al. An observational cohort study of Chlamydia trachomatis treatment in pregnancy. Sex Transm Dis 2006;33(2):106–52.
38. McLean CA, Stoner BP, Workowski KA. Treatment of lymphogranuloma vene-reum. Clin Infect Dis 2007;44(Suppl 3):S147–52.

Trichomoniasis
The "Neglected" Sexually Transmitted Disease

Elissa Meites, MD, MPH

KEYWORDS

- *Trichomonas vaginalis* • Vaginitis • Urethritis • Nucleic acid amplification tests
- Nitroimidazoles • Sexually transmitted disease

KEY POINTS

- Although *Trichomonas vaginalis* is the most prevalent curable sexually transmitted infection, it has been considered a "neglected" parasitic infection, due to limited knowledge of its sequelae and associated costs.
- Newly available diagnostic methods, including nucleic acid amplification tests, may improve the ability to identify trichomoniasis in the clinical setting.
- Infections usually can be cured with a single oral dose of a nitroimidazole antimicrobial (eg, metronidazole or tinidazole). Allergy and antimicrobial resistance are of concern, given the lack of effective treatment alternatives.
- Prevention approaches include condoms and treatment for all sex partners.

INTRODUCTION

Trichomoniasis is a sexually transmitted disease (STD) caused by the parasite *Trichomonas vaginalis* (**Fig. 1**). Although this infection is common in the United States and worldwide, it has been considered a "neglected" parasitic infection, due to limited knowledge of its sequelae and associated costs.

EPIDEMIOLOGY

T vaginalis infection is the most prevalent nonviral sexually transmitted infection:

- In the United States, an estimated 3.7 million people are infected with *T vaginalis*, more than chlamydia and gonorrhea combined.[1]

Disclosures: None.

The findings and conclusions in this report are those of the author and do not necessarily represent the official position of the CDC.

Division of STD Prevention, National Center for HIV, Viral Hepatitis, STD, and TB Prevention, Centers for Disease Control and Prevention, 1600 Clifton Road Northeast, MS E-02, Atlanta, GA 30333, USA

E-mail address: emeites@cdc.gov

Infect Dis Clin N Am 27 (2013) 755–764
http://dx.doi.org/10.1016/j.idc.2013.06.003
0891-5520/13/$ – see front matter Published by Elsevier Inc.

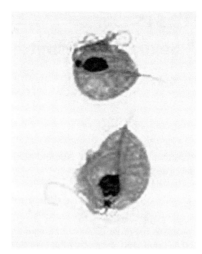

Fig. 1. *Trichomonas vaginalis* parasites.

- There are an estimated 1.1 million new *T vaginalis* infections annually in the United States.[1]
- About 3% of the United States population is believed to carry *T vaginalis* infection.[2]

Health disparities by sex, age, and race are prominent in the epidemiology of *T vaginalis*:

- Infections are believed to be more common among women, with an estimated 16 infected women for every 10 infected men.[3]
- Infections are more common with increasing age, with prevalence peaking above 11% among women aged 40 years and older.[2,4]
- Infections are more common among certain racial and ethnic groups, affecting an estimated 13.3% of black women and 1.8% of Hispanic women, compared with 1.3% of white women in the United States.[2]

Particularly high prevalences of *T vaginalis* infection have been detected among incarcerated men and women (up to 32%)[5] and patients at STD clinics (up to 17%).[6] In addition, incident *T vaginalis* infections are up to twice as common among individuals infected with the human immunodeficiency virus (HIV).[7,8] By contrast, studies among men who have sex with men have found low prevalences of *T vaginalis* infection.[9,10]

PATHOPHYSIOLOGY

The *T vaginalis* parasite is a single-celled protozoan with 4 flagella at one end. Under a microscope, these flagella may be seen propelling the parasite. Infection may produce local inflammation as parasites adhere to mucosal tissue. *T vaginalis* parasites can infect both women and men, and are passed readily between sex partners, usually during penile-vaginal sex.[11]

T vaginalis thrives in certain moist areas of the body:

- Urethra, male or female
- Vagina
- Vulva

These parasites do not commonly infect the hands, mouth, or rectum. *T vaginalis* parasites require a human host and do not affect any other animals. Although these parasites might be able to survive for a few minutes in damp environments outside the human body, there have been no proven cases of transmission via shared baths, toilets, or towels.

Clinical signs and symptoms of trichomoniasis are variable and may include:

- Itching or irritation
- Local erythema
- Burning sensation during urination or ejaculation
- Vaginal or urethral frothy discharge that may be any color but is classically yellow/green and malodorous
- None, because 70% to 85% of infected persons are asymptomatic[2,12]

Initial symptoms may develop within 5 to 28 days. However, untreated infections can last for months to years, and symptoms might occur at any time.[13]

DIAGNOSIS

Several newly available diagnostic assays may improve the ability to identify *T vaginalis* infections in comparison with traditional methods. Available diagnostic methods include the following:

- APTIMA Trichomonas vaginalis assay, a highly sensitive nucleic acid amplification test (NAAT)
- OSOM Trichomonas Rapid Test, a dipstick that can be used at the point of care
- Affirm VPIII, a nucleic acid probe that assesses 3 microbial causes of vaginitis
- Wet mount microscopy, a common low-cost test with poor sensitivity
- Culture, the traditional gold-standard method

The first highly sensitive NAAT was cleared by the United States Food and Drug Administration (FDA) in 2011. The APTIMA Trichomonas vaginalis assay (Hologic Gen-Probe, San Diego, CA) can be used on vaginal, endocervical, or urine specimens. This assay uses transcription-mediated amplification with a clinical sensitivity of 95% to 100% and specificity of 95% to 100%, producing results within hours.[14–16] Although the assay has not been cleared by the FDA for use with penile swabs or urine from men, some laboratories have procedures in place to use the components as an in-house test. This test method may be particularly appealing for laboratories that use the same platform to conduct chlamydia and gonorrhea screening tests, as this assay can be run on the same specimen.

Same-day tests cleared by the FDA for the diagnosis of trichomoniasis include the OSOM Trichomonas Rapid Test (Sekisui Diagnostics, Framingham, MA), and the Affirm VPIII (Becton Dickinson, San Jose, CA). The OSOM is a CLIA (Clinical Laboratory Improvement Amendments)-waived dipstick assay that can provide results at the point of care within approximately 10 minutes. It is an antigen-detection test that uses immunochromatographic capillary flow technology on vaginal swabs with sensitivity of 82% to 95% and specificity of 97% to 100%.[15,17] The Affirm VPIII evaluates causes of vaginitis including *T vaginalis*, *Gardnerella vaginalis*, and *Candida albicans*. The probe for *T. vaginalis* uses nucleic acid probe-hybridization with sensitivity of 63% and specificity of 99.9%, and takes about 45 minutes in the laboratory.[16] Neither the OSOM nor the Affirm VPIII has been approved by the FDA for use on male specimens.

Traditionally, the most common method used to identify *T vaginalis* has been wet mount (saline) microscopy, whereby clinician or laboratory operator examines a mixture of saline and genital fluid (eg, vaginal discharge) on a glass slide under a microscope, attempting to identify the characteristic motile parasites of T vaginalis. Advantages of this method include low cost and immediate results, but major disadvantages are variability in skill and generally poor sensitivity, even with experienced observers (51%–65%), especially for specimens from males.[15,18] Wet mount specimens should be examined as soon as possible after collection for best results, as sensitivity declines rapidly after specimen preparation.[19]

The traditional gold standard is culture, a highly specific method for identifying T vaginalis, but disadvantages include the need for specialized equipment including transport and culture media, and a delayed time to result. Cultures may be inoculated with a variety of specimen types from men or women, including genital secretions, semen, or urine.

Neither traditional nor liquid-based Papanicolaou tests (Pap smears) are considered appropriate diagnostic or screening tests for trichomoniasis because of their poor sensitivity.[20,21] However, the specificity of liquid-based cytology for T vaginalis is high.[22,23] When the parasite is an incidental finding, treatment is usually indicated, although at the discretion of the clinician for asymptomatic patients.[24]

The main reasons to check for T vaginalis are:

- To reduce symptoms by treating disease
- To reduce potential sequelae by curing infection

Diagnostic testing is recommended for all women presenting with symptoms of trichomoniasis (ie, vaginitis or vaginal discharge). For men with symptoms of trichomoniasis (ie, urethritis), trichomoniasis is less likely to be the cause, but testing could be considered if initial workup does not yield an alternative diagnosis. If diagnostic tests appropriate for use in males are not available, therapy for trichomoniasis can be considered as a second-line therapy for nongonococcal urethritis, recommended if the initial empiric regimens for nongonococcal urethritis (usually azithromycin or doxycycline) fail.[25,26]

Screening for T vaginalis infection is recommended for HIV-infected women at entry to care and at least annually thereafter.[24] Screening may be considered for asymptomatic persons receiving care in high-prevalence settings such as STD clinics and correctional facilities, as well as those at high risk of infection or disease (eg, persons with new or multiple sex partners or history of any STD). Decisions about screening may be informed by local, regional, or national epidemiology of T vaginalis infection.

The benefits and effectiveness of screening asymptomatic men are still unknown. In the absence of scientific evidence that symptoms or sequelae could be reduced by treatment of T vaginalis, testing and screening are not recommended for men.

CLINICAL MANAGEMENT

Infections usually can be cured with 5-nitroimidazole antimicrobials, which are the only class of medications approved by the FDA for treatment of trichomoniasis. First-line therapy consists of either metronidazole (Flagyl) or tinidazole (Tindamax), 2 g in a single dose, given either orally or intravenously (Box 1). These medications are widely available and fairly inexpensive, particularly metronidazole. Tinidazole has a longer half-life and achieves a higher genitourinary tract drug level than metronidazole, but it is more expensive. Topically applied antimicrobials such as metronidazole gel have high failure rates (>50%). Treating patients and all sex partners can cure infection, reduce symptoms, and reduce transmission.[24]

> **Box 1**
> **Recommended regimens for treating trichomoniasis, according to the 2010 STD treatment guidelines of the Centers for Disease Control and Prevention**
>
> *Recommended Regimens*
>
> Metronidazole: 2 g orally in a single dose
>
> OR
>
> Tinidazole: 2 g orally in a single dose
>
> *Alternative Regimen*
>
> Metronidazole: 500 mg orally twice a day for 7 days
>
> *From* Workowski KA, Berman S, Centers for Disease Control and Prevention. Sexually transmitted disease treatment guidelines, 2010. MMWR 2010;59(RR-12):1–110.

Allergy and antimicrobial resistance are of concern, given the lack of effective alternatives to nitroimidazoles.

Allergic reactions should be distinguished from potential side effects of nitroimidazole medication, which can include disulfiram-like reactions with flushing. True hypersensitivity reactions occur occasionally and may include urticaria, pruritus, facial edema, erythema, and gastrointestinal or other symptoms; true anaphylaxis is rare. Desensitization therapy according to a 14-step incremental dosing protocol can be effective in the management of trichomoniasis for patients with nitroimidazole hypersensitivity.[27]

When trichomoniasis does not respond to standard therapy, considerations include reinfection versus refractory disease. If reinfection from an untreated partner is excluded, patients can be treated with the alternative regimen of metronidazole, 500 mg orally twice daily for 7 days. For disease refractory to both recommended and alternative regimens, treatment with tinidazole or metronidazole, at least 2 g orally for 5 to 7 days, can be considered. If none of these regimens are effective, consultation with a specialist may be helpful, ideally including antimicrobial susceptibility testing to determine the resistance profile of the parasite.[24]

Antimicrobial resistance is an emerging issue of concern, given the lack of effective alternative treatments for trichomoniasis. In vitro, approximately 4% of *T vaginalis* parasites exhibit some degree of resistance to metronidazole, although correlation with clinical outcomes remains unclear. Tinidazole may be more active against *T vaginalis* isolates that demonstrate resistance. Susceptibility testing and consultation are available from the Centers for Disease Control and Prevention.[28]

ADVERSE OUTCOMES

Traditionally there has been little appreciation of adverse outcomes associated with *T vaginalis* infection, as trichomoniasis rarely results in hospitalizations or deaths. An analysis of the direct medical costs of incident sexually transmitted infections in the United States estimated that 1.1 million new cases of trichomoniasis per year cost only US$24 million.[29] In that analysis, the lifetime cost per case of trichomoniasis, at $22, was the least expensive of any sexually transmitted infection, based on the assumption that persons with untreated *T vaginalis* infections do not incur any costs.[29] However, various recent studies have increased appreciation for the possibility that even asymptomatic *T vaginalis* infections can be linked to a variety of other health problems. Conditions shown to be associated with *T vaginalis* infection include:

- Increased risk of HIV acquisition and transmission[30]
- Increased prevalence of other sexually transmitted infections[31]
- Adverse outcomes of pregnancy (eg, preterm delivery)[32]
- Pelvic inflammatory disease among HIV-infected women[33]

T vaginalis infection was an independent risk factor for HIV in several recent studies, which found it to significantly increase the risk of acquiring HIV by 2 to 3 times.[30,34,35] Furthermore, maternal *T vaginalis* infection in an HIV-infected woman nearly doubles the risk of vertical transmission of HIV to the infant.[36] Interestingly, HIV-infected women are less likely to shed HIV vaginally after receiving treatment for trichomoniasis.[37,38] However, there are no data to show that treating *T vaginalis* can reverse the increased risks of HIV acquisition or transmission.

In a nationally representative study, 6 other sexually transmitted infections (chlamydia, gonorrhea, herpes simplex virus type 1, herpes simplex virus type 2, syphilis, and HIV) all were more common among women with a positive test for *T vaginalis*.[31]

Pregnant women who are infected with *T vaginalis* are more likely to deliver preterm infants, with correspondingly low birth weights.[32,39] In addition, ecological studies have suggested links between maternal trichomoniasis during pregnancy and having a child with intellectual disability or attention deficit/hyperactivity disorder, although the mechanism of association remains unclear.[40,41] Among HIV-infected women, those with concomitant *T vaginalis* infection are at a significantly increased risk for pelvic inflammatory disease.[33]

Researchers have also investigated possible associations between trichomoniasis and other conditions, such as male and female infertility[42,43] or prostate cancer,[44,45] but these relationships remain uncertain.

Additional studies considering the aforementioned sequelae would produce higher estimates of the costs of *T vaginalis* infections. For example, a mathematical model of HIV infections attributable to trichomoniasis in the United States estimated that each year, 746 new HIV cases among women could be attributed to trichomoniasis, at a lifetime cost of approximately $167 million.[46]

SPECIAL CONSIDERATIONS
HIV

HIV-infected individuals should be screened at least annually for *T vaginalis* infections, given the high prevalence,[7] increased risk of pelvic inflammatory disease,[33] and ability of nitroimidazole treatment to reduce HIV viral shedding.[37] Those who are found to be infected with *T vaginalis* may benefit from an extended course of treatment. A study comparing the single-dose regimen with the 7-day alternative regimen of metronidazole found that HIV-infected women receiving the longer treatment course had a reduced risk of remaining infected with *T vaginalis,* both at test of cure and 3 months later.[47]

Pregnancy and Breastfeeding

Screening and treatment for *T vaginalis* infections can be considered for pregnant women, although it remains unclear whether such intervention improves outcomes for pregnant women and their infants. Metronidazole is safe for use during any stage of pregnancy or breastfeeding, although tinidazole should be avoided because of a theoretical risk to the infant.[24,48]

Children

T vaginalis colonization of the neonate has been known to occur during delivery and usually self-resolves within weeks without sequelae. Treatment is not usually necessary. In a child, *T vaginalis* infection is suspicious for sexual abuse.

PREVENTION

Approaches to preventing trichomoniasis include:

- Abstaining from sex
- Using condoms
- Ensuring that all sex partners receive adequate treatment
- Refraining from douching

STDs, including trichomoniasis, can be avoided by abstaining entirely from sex. Among sexually active individuals, however, a more realistic approach may be to use condoms consistently and correctly.[49]

All sex partners of a person diagnosed with *T vaginalis* infection should be notified promptly and treated appropriately before resuming sexual activity. Patient-delivered partner therapy has been found to be as effective as standard notification, and is an option in states where this strategy is permissible.[50,51]

Douching is not effective in reducing trichomoniasis; on the contrary, this practice may be a risk factor for *T vaginalis* and other sexually transmitted infections.[2,52]

CONTROVERSIES

Neither trichomoniasis nor *T vaginalis* infection is a nationally notifiable condition in the United States.[53] Furthermore, neither the infection nor the disease is currently reportable to the health department of any state. Although the frequency, communicability, and associated health disparities have been clearly identified, consistent data are still lacking regarding severity of infection, preventability of associated adverse events, and costs. Finally, there has been little interest in this infection among members of the general public.[53]

SUMMARY

Although *T vaginalis* infection is quite common, and usually curable with a widely available and fairly inexpensive medication, a lack of public awareness makes trichomoniasis a "neglected" STD. Disparities in the prevalence of infection by sex, age, race/ethnicity, and setting should be recognized. The emergence of antimicrobial resistance and lack of alternative treatments is of concern. Additional data regarding the severity and costs of infection, as well as evidence that treatment of *T vaginalis* can prevent associated conditions, could lead to wider recognition of this infection in the future.

REFERENCES

1. Satterwhite CL, Torrone E, Meites E, et al. Sexually transmitted infections among US women and men: prevalence and incidence estimates, 2008. Sex Transm Dis 2013;40(3):187–93 [Systemic review or meta-analysis].
2. Sutton M, Sternberg M, Koumans EH, et al. The prevalence of *Trichomonas vaginalis* infection among reproductive-age women in the United States, 2001–2004. Clin Infect Dis 2007;45(10):1319–26.

3. Miller WC, Swygard H, Hobbs MM, et al. The prevalence of trichomoniasis in young adults in the United States. Sex Transm Dis 2005;32(10):593–8.

4. Ginocchio CC, Chapin K, Smith JS, et al. Prevalence of *Trichomonas vaginalis* and coinfection with *Chlamydia trachomatis* and *Neisseria gonorrhoeae* in the United States as determined by the Aptima Trichomonas vaginalis nucleic acid amplification assay. J Clin Microbiol 2012;50(8):2601–8.

5. Freeman AH, Katz KA, Pandori MW, et al. Prevalence and correlates of *Trichomonas vaginalis* among incarcerated persons assessed using a highly sensitive molecular assay. Sex Transm Dis 2010;37(3):165–8.

6. Schwebke JR, Hook EW. High rates of *Trichomonas vaginalis* among men attending a sexually transmitted diseases clinic: implications for screening and urethritis management. J Infect Dis 2003;188(3):465–8.

7. Cu-Uvin S, Ko H, Jamieson DJ, et al. Prevalence, incidence, and persistence or recurrence of trichomoniasis among human immunodeficiency virus (HIV)-positive women and among HIV-negative women at high risk for HIV infection. Clin Infect Dis 2002;34(10):1406–11.

8. Mullins TL, Rudy BJ, Wilson CM, et al. Incidence of sexually transmitted infections in HIV-infected and HIV-uninfected adolescents in the USA. Int J STD AIDS 2013;24(2):123–7.

9. Mayer KH, Bush T, Henry K, et al. Ongoing sexually transmitted disease acquisition and risk-taking behavior among US HIV-infected patients in primary care: implications for prevention interventions. Sex Transm Dis 2012;39(1):1–7.

10. Kelley CF, Rosenberg ES, O'Hara BM, et al. Prevalence of urethral *Trichomonas vaginalis* in black and white men who have sex with men. Sex Transm Dis 2012;39(9):739.

11. Seña AC, Miller WC, Hobbs MM, et al. *Trichomonas vaginalis* infection in male sexual partners: implications for diagnosis, treatment, and prevention. Clin Infect Dis 2007;44(1):13–22.

12. Peterman TA, Tian LH, Metcalf CA, et al. High incidence of new sexually transmitted infections in the year following a sexually transmitted infection: a case for rescreening. Ann Intern Med 2006;145(8):564–72.

13. Bachmann LH, Hobbs MM, Seña AC, et al. *Trichomonas vaginalis* genital infections: progress and challenges. Clin Infect Dis 2011;53(Suppl 3):S160–72.

14. Schwebke JR, Hobbs MM, Taylor SN, et al. Molecular testing for *Trichomonas vaginalis* in women: results from a prospective U.S. clinical trial. J Clin Microbiol 2011;49(12):4106–11.

15. Huppert JS, Mortensen JE, Reed JL, et al. Rapid antigen testing compares favorably with transcription-mediated amplification assay for the detection of *Trichomonas vaginalis* in young women. Clin Infect Dis 2007;45(2):194–8.

16. Andrea SB, Chapin KC. Comparison of Aptima Trichomonas vaginalis transcription-mediated amplification assay and BD affirm VPIII for detection of *T. vaginalis* in symptomatic women: performance parameters and epidemiological implications. J Clin Microbiol 2011;49(3):866–9.

17. Campbell L, Woods V, Lloyd T, et al. Evaluation of the OSOM Trichomonas rapid test versus wet preparation examination for detection of *Trichomonas vaginalis* vaginitis in specimens from women with a low prevalence of infection. J Clin Microbiol 2008;46(10):3467–9.

18. Nye MB, Schwebke JR, Body BA. Comparison of APTIMA Trichomonas vaginalis transcription-mediated amplification to wet mount microscopy, culture, and polymerase chain reaction for diagnosis of trichomoniasis in men and women. Am J Obstet Gynecol 2009;200(2):188.e1–7.

19. Stoner KA, Rabe LK, Meyn LA, et al. Survival of *Trichomonas vaginalis* in wet preparation and on wet mount. Sex Transm Infect 2013;89(6):485–8.
20. Lobo TT, Feijo G, Carvalho SE, et al. A comparative evaluation of the Papanicolaou test for the diagnosis of trichomoniasis. Sex Transm Dis 2003;30(9):694–9.
21. Lara-Torre E, Pinkerton JS. Accuracy of detection of *Trichomonas vaginalis* organisms on a liquid-based Papanicolaou smear. Am J Obstet Gynecol 2003; 188(2):354–6.
22. Noel JC, Engohan-Aloghe C. Morphologic criteria associated with *Trichomonas vaginalis* in liquid-based cytology. Acta Cytol 2010;54(4):582–6.
23. Aslan DL, Gulbahce HE, Stelow EB, et al. The diagnosis of *Trichomonas vaginalis* in liquid-based Pap tests: correlation with PCR. Diagn Cytopathol 2005;32(6): 341–4.
24. Workowski KA, Berman S, Centers for Disease Control and Prevention. Sexually transmitted diseases treatment guidelines, 2010. MMWR Recomm Rep 2010; 59(RR-12):1–110 [Systemic review or meta-analysis].
25. Schwebke JR, Rompalo A, Taylor S, et al. Re-evaluating the treatment of nongonococcal urethritis: emphasizing emerging pathogens—a randomized clinical trial. Clin Infect Dis 2011;52(2):163–70.
26. Seña AC, Lensing S, Rompalo A, et al. *Chlamydia trachomatis, Mycoplasma genitalium*, and *Trichomonas vaginalis* infections in men with nongonococcal urethritis: predictors and persistence after therapy. J Infect Dis 2012;206(3):357–65.
27. Helms DJ, Mosure DJ, Secor WE, et al. Management of *Trichomonas vaginalis* in women with suspected metronidazole hypersensitivity. Am J Obstet Gynecol 2008;198(4):370.e1–7.
28. Kirkcaldy RD, Augostini P, Asbel LE, et al. *Trichomonas vaginalis* antimicrobial drug resistance in 6 US cities, STD Surveillance Network, 2009-2010. Emerg Infect Dis 2012;18(6):939–43.
29. Owusu-Edusei K Jr, Chesson HW, Gift TL, et al. The estimated direct medical cost of selected sexually transmitted infections in the United States, 2008. Sex Transm Dis 2013;40(3):197–201 [Systemic review or meta-analysis].
30. Hughes JP, Baeten JM, Lingappa JR, et al. Determinants of per-coital-act HIV-1 infectivity among African HIV-1-serodiscordant couples. J Infect Dis 2012; 205(3):358–65.
31. Allsworth JE, Ratner JA, Peipert JF. Trichomoniasis and other sexually transmitted infections: results from the 2001-2004 National Health and Nutrition Examination Surveys. Sex Transm Dis 2009;36(12):738–44.
32. Cotch MF, Pastorek JG 2nd, Nugent RP, et al. *Trichomonas vaginalis* associated with low birth weight and preterm delivery. The Vaginal Infections and Prematurity Study Group. Sex Transm Dis 1997;24(6):353–60.
33. Moodley P, Wilkinson D, Connolly C, et al. *Trichomonas vaginalis* is associated with pelvic inflammatory disease in women infected with human immunodeficiency virus. Clin Infect Dis 2002;34(4):519–22.
34. Mavedzenge SN, Pol BV, Cheng H, et al. Epidemiological synergy of *Trichomonas vaginalis* and HIV in Zimbabwean and South African women. Sex Transm Dis 2010;37(7):460–6.
35. Van Der Pol B, Kwok C, Pierre-Louis B, et al. *Trichomonas vaginalis* infection and human immunodeficiency virus acquisition in African women. J Infect Dis 2008; 197(4):548–54.
36. Gumbo FZ, Duri K, Kandawasvika GQ, et al. Risk factors of HIV vertical transmission in a cohort of women under a PMTCT program at three peri-urban clinics in a resource-poor setting. J Perinatol 2010;30(11):717–23.

37. Kissinger P, Amedee A, Clark RA, et al. *Trichomonas vaginalis* treatment reduces vaginal HIV-1 shedding. Sex Transm Dis 2009;36(1):11–6.

38. Anderson BL, Firnhaber C, Liu T, et al. Effect of trichomoniasis therapy on genital HIV viral burden among African women. Sex Transm Dis 2012;39(8):638–42.

39. Mann JR, McDermott S, Gill T. Sexually transmitted infection is associated with increased risk of preterm birth in South Carolina women insured by Medicaid. J Matern Fetal Neonatal Med 2010;23(6):563–8.

40. Mann JR, McDermott S, Barnes TL, et al. Trichomoniasis in pregnancy and mental retardation in children. Ann Epidemiol 2009;19(12):891–9.

41. Mann JR, McDermott S. Are maternal genitourinary infection and pre-eclampsia associated with ADHD in school-aged children? J Atten Disord 2011;15(8): 667–73.

42. Benchimol M, de Andrade Rosa I, da Silva Fontes R, et al. *Trichomonas* adhere and phagocytose sperm cells: adhesion seems to be a prominent stage during interaction. Parasitol Res 2008;102(4):597–604.

43. Sherman KJ, Daling JR, Weiss NS. Sexually transmitted diseases and tubal infertility. Sex Transm Dis 1987;14(1):12–6.

44. Sutcliffe S, Alderete JF, Till C, et al. Trichomonosis and subsequent risk of prostate cancer in the Prostate Cancer Prevention Trial. Int J Cancer 2009;124(9):2082–7.

45. Stark JR, Judson G, Alderete JF, et al. Prospective study of *Trichomonas vaginalis* infection and prostate cancer incidence and mortality: Physicians' Health Study. J Natl Cancer Inst 2009;101(20):1406–11.

46. Chesson HW, Blandford JM, Pinkerton SD. Estimates of the annual number and cost of new HIV infections among women attributable to trichomoniasis in the United States. Sex Transm Dis 2004;31(9):547–51.

47. Kissinger P, Mena L, Levison J, et al. A randomized treatment trial: single versus 7-day dose of metronidazole for the treatment of *Trichomonas vaginalis* among HIV-infected women. J Acquir Immune Defic Syndr 2010;55(5):565–71.

48. Gülmezoglu AM, Azhar M. Interventions for trichomoniasis in pregnancy. Cochrane Database Syst Rev 2011;(5):CD000220. [Systemic review or meta-analysis].

49. Crosby RA, Charnigo RA, Weathers C, et al. Condom effectiveness against non-viral sexually transmitted infections: a prospective study using electronic daily diaries. Sex Transm Infect 2012;88(7):484–9.

50. Kissinger P, Schmidt N, Mohammed H, et al. Patient-delivered partner treatment for *Trichomonas vaginalis* infection: a randomized controlled trial. Sex Transm Dis 2006;33(7):445–50.

51. Schwebke JR, Desmond RA. A randomized controlled trial of partner notification methods for prevention of trichomoniasis in women. Sex Transm Dis 2010;37(6): 392–6.

52. Tsai CS, Shepherd BE, Vermund SH. Does douching increase risk for sexually transmitted infections? A prospective study in high-risk adolescents. Am J Obstet Gynecol 2009;200(1):38.e1–8.

53. Hoots BE, Peterman TA, Torrone EA, et al. A Trich-y question: should *Trichomonas vaginalis* infection be reportable? Sex Transm Dis 2013;40(2):113–6.

HPV and HPV-Associated Diseases

Eileen F. Dunne, MD, MPH[a],*, Ina U. Park, MD, MS[b,c]

KEYWORDS

- HPV • Anogenital warts • Genital warts • HPV-associated diseases
- Cervical cancer • HPV vaccines

KEY POINTS

- Human papillomavirus (HPV) is the most common sexually transmitted infection. Most infections clear within 2 years and do not result in disease or cancer.
- HPV can cause anogenital warts, recurrent respiratory papillomatosis, oropharyngeal cancer, and a variety of anogenital cancers in men and women (including penile, anal, vaginal, vulvar, and cervical cancers).
- Effective prevention is available, including primary prevention of cancers and anogenital warts through HPV vaccination, and secondary prevention of cervical cancer through screening and treatment of precancer.
- Effective patient-applied and provider-administered treatments are available for anogenital warts.
- The burden of HPV-associated conditions/cancers is greater in specific populations, including those who are immunocompromised (eg, from human immunodeficiency virus infection or post-transplant).

BACKGROUND

Papillomaviruses are a family of DNA viruses that infect the epithelium and have a double-stranded, closed, circular genome of approximately 8 kb and a nonenveloped icosahedral capsid. Mucosal human papillomavirus (HPV) types are divided into 2 groups based on their association with cancer. Low-risk, or nononcogenic, HPV types are associated with anogenital warts and recurrent respiratory papillomatosis (RRP). Persistent infection with high-risk, or oncogenic, HPV types is the most important risk factor for the development of cancers, including cervical, penile, anal, vaginal, vulvar, and oropharyngeal cancer. Routine cervical cancer screening of women is

The findings and conclusions in this report are those of the authors and do not necessarily represent the views of CDC.

[a] Division of STD Prevention, Centers for Disease Control and Prevention, 1600 Clifton Road, MS E-02, Atlanta, GA 30030, USA; [b] Department of Family and Community Medicine, University of California San Francisco School of Medicine, 995 Potrero Avenue, Ward 83, San Francisco, CA 94110, USA; [c] California STD/HIV Prevention Training Center, 300 Frank Ogawa Plaza, Suite 520, Oakland, CA 94612, USA
* Corresponding author.
E-mail address: Dde9@cdc.gov

Infect Dis Clin N Am 27 (2013) 765–778
http://dx.doi.org/10.1016/j.idc.2013.09.001
0891-5520/13/$ – see front matter Published by Elsevier Inc.

id.theclinics.com

recommended starting at age 21 years. Prophylactic HPV vaccines are routinely recommended for boys and girls at age 11 or 12 years. Recent data from the United States and Australia strongly support that widespread vaccination and cervical cancer screening can potentially reduce the substantial burden of HPV-associated disease.

MAGNITUDE OF INFECTION/DISEASE BURDEN

HPV is the most common sexually transmitted infection. In the United States, 14 million persons acquire HPV each year and 79 million have prevalent infection[1]; most sexually active persons will have detectable HPV at least once in their lifetime. Overall annual medical costs related to HPV-associated diseases (warts, RRP, precancer, cancer) are estimated at $8 billion in the United States.[2]

The annual incidence of anogenital warts based on a systematic review of 32 studies conducted worldwide ranged from 160 to 289 cases per 100,000 persons.[3] The best estimates from the United States are from health claims databases; the incidence in one study was 1.2 cases per 1000 in women and 1.1 cases per 1000 in men.[4] Anogenital wart incidence is highest in women aged 20 to 24 years, and men aged 25 to 29 years.[4–6] Based on these data, an estimated 340,000 new anogenital wart cases occur in the United States each year.[2,4] The burden of RRP is difficult to assess because no routine surveillance is performed and it is a rare condition; however, based on one evaluation in urban settings, an estimated 80 to 1500 cases of juvenile-onset RRP occurred in 1999.[7]

The most recent estimates for HPV-associated cancers in the United States are from the Annual Report to the Nation using data from the Surveillance Epidemiology and End Results Program and the National Program of Cancer Registries.[8] An estimated 34,788 new HPV-associated cancers in men and women occurred in 2009, including cervical, anal, penile, oropharyngeal, vaginal, and vulvar cancers, with oropharyngeal (13,000) and cervical (11,400) being the most prevalent. A substantial proportion of these cancers are attributable to HPV 16/18 and are potentially vaccine-preventable, ranging from approximately 60% for oropharyngeal cancer to 85% for anal cancer.[9]

The burden of HPV-associated conditions/cancers is greater in immunocompromised persons, such as those with human immunodeficiency virus (HIV) infection or who have undergone transplant. Using data from 13 cohort studies in the United States and Canada, a recent study estimated that the rate ratio for anal cancer in HIV-infected men and HIV-infected men who have sex with men (MSM) compared with HIV-negative men was 26.7 and 80.3, respectively.[10] The incidence of HPV-associated warts and cancer has not decreased with the advent of effective antiretroviral therapy (ART) for HIV. One study found that the incidence of anal cancer increased 6-fold between pre-ART and post-ART periods, from 8.5 per 100,000 person years in 1992–1996, to 53.2 per 100,000 person years in 2005–2008.[11] A study of anogenital warts found that the unadjusted cumulative incidence was 9.3% (95% confidence interval [CI], 6.3–12.2) in HIV-uninfected women, 28.4% (95% CI, 21.7–34.5) in HIV-infected women who initiated ART, and 25.1% (95% CI, 18.4–31.2) in HIV-infected women who did not initiate ART.[12]

EPIDEMIOLOGY OF HPV: TRANSMISSION AND NATURAL HISTORY

HPV infection often occurs shortly after initiation of sexual activity; in one study, the cumulative incidence of any HPV infection at 1 year among college-aged women after sexual debut was 28.5%, and increased to almost 50% by 3 years.[13] Even persons with 1 lifetime sex partner are at risk for infection; one study found that 14.3% of women aged 18 to 25 years with 1 lifetime sex partner had HPV infection, increasing to 22.3% with 2 lifetime sex partners, and 31.5% with more than 3 lifetime partners.[14] Most HPV infections are transient, with 90% of men and women typically clearing infection within 2 years.[13,15–17] Among young women, peak prevalence of HPV occurs at 20 to 24 years of age.[18] However, among men, the prevalence of HPV remains steady through the fifth and sixth decades.[19,20]

HPV is often transmitted through vaginal or anal intercourse; transmission can also occur through oral-genital or genital-genital contact. A study of young women who reported no previous sexual intercourse and had other sexual activity, such as genital-genital or genital-oral contact, found that the 24-month cumulative incidence of infection was 7.9% (95% CI, 3.5–17.1).[13] In one study, HPV was detected in 45.5% of subjects (10 of 22) before first vaginal sex, and 7 of these 10 subjects reported noncoital behaviors that may have resulted in genital transmission.[21] These findings are supported by the observation that women who report only sexual experience with other women have a risk of genital HPV infection similar to their heterosexual counterparts.[22]

HPV transmission occurs frequently between sexual partners. Multiple studies of heterosexual couples show higher rates of transmission from women to men than from men to women. Rates of transmission range from 3.5 to 187.5 transmission events per 100 person months, with the highest rates observed in studies in which sampling was performed 24 hours after vaginal intercourse.[23–25] A meta-analysis of 33 studies examining concordance of HPV types among couples showed 25.5% concordance for at least 1 HPV type, although concordance for 1 or more types was as high as 62.5% when both partners were HPV-positive.[26]

NATURAL HISTORY OF HPV-ASSOCIATED DISEASES

Infection with low-risk HPV types can lead to genital warts; 90% of genital warts are caused by HPV 6 and 11. Studies of HPV infection and anogenital warts show that the median time to development of warts after a new infection is 3 to 10 months, although this can range up to as long as 47 months.[27–29] In one study, the 36-month cumulative incidence of genital warts among women with incident HPV 6 or 11 infection was 64.2% (95% CI, 50.7%–77.4%).[30] Genital warts are generally benign and resolve within 6 months (with or without treatment). However, a large proportion (≈30%) of genital warts recur, which can result in frequent office visits, sometimes costly and debilitating treatment, and substantial psychosocial burden.[2,31] Rare cases have been reported of giant condyloma acuminatum of Bushke and Lowenstein, a slow-growing and destructive condyloma caused by HPV 6 or 11 infection that does not metastasize but may have a foci of squamous cell carcinoma.[32] This condition most commonly occurs among immunocompromised individuals, including patients with HIV or those who have undergone solid organ transplant.

HPV often leads to low-grade cervical disease. The prognosis for these women is excellent. Cervical intraepithelial neoplasia (CIN) 1 (a low-grade histologic change, often considered just a histologic manifestation of HPV infection) usually clears spontaneously (60% of cases) and rarely progresses to cancer (1%).[33,34] Therefore, the recommendation for management for these lesions is to repeat cytology/histology rather than treat. Persistent infection with oncogenic HPV types can lead to high-grade cervical disease (CIN 2, 3) and cervical cancer. A lower percentage of high-grade lesions spontaneously clear (40% for CIN 2 and 33% for CIN 3), and a higher percentage progress to cancer if not treated (5% for CIN 2 and >12% for

CIN 3).[33,34] Treatment of these lesions prevents the progression to invasive cancer. The prognosis for cervical cancers may depend on the stage at diagnosis, size of the tumor, and age of the woman.

The pathogenesis of anal cancer is thought to be similar to cervical cancer, beginning with persistent infection with oncogenic HPV types, and progressing to precancerous changes and cancer. A systematic review of HPV type distribution in anal cancer found that 72% of anal cancers were attributable to HPV 16/18, similar to that reported for cervical cancer.[35] However, the natural history of anal cancer precursors, such as high-grade anal intraepithelial neoplasia (AIN-2,3), is not well understood. No prospective data are available on regression rates of high-grade AIN or progression of high-grade AIN to anal cancer. Prognosis for anal cancer depends on the size of the primary tumor and nodal status. For stage I cancer, prognosis is favorable, with a 5-year survival rate of approximately 70%.[36]

CLINICAL FEATURES

Infection with anogenital HPV is usually asymptomatic, and infection usually resolves without consequences. Screening is not routinely recommended other than for cervical cancer (**Table 1**). When disease does occur, one of the most common clinical manifestations of HPV is anogenital warts. Genital warts appear as small papules, or flat, smooth, or pedunculated lesions. Sometimes they can be soft, pink, or white cauliflower-like sessile growths on moist mucosal surfaces (condyloma acuminatum), or keratotic lesions on squamous epithelium of the skin with a thick, horny layer. If anogenital warts are detected, some experts recommend conducting a complete anogenital examination. Detection of genital warts is not a reason to recommend more frequent cervical cancer screening, because the HPV types that cause genital warts are different from those that cause cancer.

Cervical lesions caused by HPV (CIN) are often not visible with speculum examination or even colposcopic magnification and application of acetic acid or Lugol's iodine. Colposcopic features of high-grade CIN lesions when they occur include sharply demarcated margins, dense acetowhitening or gray coloration, vascular abnormalities (punctate vessels and mosaic patterns), and strong nonstaining patterns after application of iodine.

Anal lesions can occasionally be visualized with the naked eye on simple anoscopy, but most often require magnification and application of acetic acid or Lugol's iodine, also called *high-resolution anoscopy* (HRA). HRA features of high-grade AIN are generally similar to colposcopic features of high-grade CIN.

SCREENING AND DIAGNOSTIC APPROACHES

Anogenital warts are usually diagnosed through visual inspection. This diagnosis can then be confirmed with biopsy, which is indicated if lesions are atypical, such as those that are pigmented, indurated, fixed to underlying tissue, bleeding, or ulcerated. Biopsy may also be indicated if the diagnosis is uncertain, or the lesions do not respond to standard therapy, or the disease worsens during therapy. Biopsy should be considered in these circumstances, especially in patients who are immunocompromised (including those with HIV infection). Providers should test patients with a new diagnosis of anogenital warts for HIV infection and other sexually transmitted infections. Anogenital warts can mimic other conditions, including molluscum contagiosum, condyloma lata (a sign of secondary syphilis), squamous intraepithelial lesions, and other skin conditions.

Table 1
Screening guidelines for women at average risk for cervical cancer and for women with HIV infection

	Average Risk[a]	HIV Infection
Initiating screening	Begin screening at age 21 y	Consider screening within 1 y of initiation of sexual activity, regardless of age
	Women aged <21 y should not be screened regardless of age of sexual initiation or risk factors	HIV-positive women should be screened with a Papanicolau test at 6-mo intervals in the first year after HIV-diagnosis
Annual screening	Not recommended for any age group.	Annual screening is recommended
Screening method suggested intervals	Age 21–29 y: cytology alone every 3 y, HPV co-testing should not be used	Cytology alone every year
	Age 30–35 y: cytology alone every 3 y, or cytology with HPV co-testing every 5 y	
When to stop screening	Age >65 y with an adequate screening history	Lifelong screening is recommended
Screening posthysterectomy	If cervix removed and no history of precancer or cancer, discontinue screening	No national recommendations exist regarding need for screening posthysterectomy
	If supracervical hysterectomy, should continue screening according to guidelines	
Screening of vaccinated women	Continue screening according to age specific recommendations	Continue annual screening

[a] These recommendations do not apply to women with a history of high-grade cervical intraepithelial neoplasia (CIN 2 or 3) or cervical cancer, with in utero exposure to diethylstilbestrol, who are immunocompromised, or who are HIV-positive.

Data from Centers for Disease Control and Prevention-Division of Cancer Prevention and Control. Cervical Cancer Screening Guidelines for Average-Risk Women. Available at: http://www.cdc.gov/cancer/cervical/pdf/guidelines.pdf. Accessed August 3, 2012; and Panel on Opportunistic Infections in HIV-Infected Adults and Adolescents. Guidelines for the prevention and treatment of opportunistic infections in HIV-infected adults and adolescents: recommendations from the Centers for Disease Control and Prevention, the National Institutes of Health, and the HIV Medicine Association of the Infectious Diseases Society of America. Available at: http://aidsinfo.nih.gov/contentfiles/lvguidelines/adult_oi.pdf. Accessed August 3, 2013.

Cervical lesions are detected through routine cervical cancer screening. All women who are sexually active, including those who have sex only with women, are at risk for CIN and cervical cancer. Cervical cancer screening guidelines for the general population were recently revised in 2012.[37] **Table 1** compares screening guidelines for average-risk women versus those with HIV infection. For average-risk women, screening should begin at age 21 years and continue at 3- to 5-year intervals (depending on age and screening test used) until 65 years of age. Because of the increased risk of cervical cancer in women with HIV infection, screening should begin 1 year after sexual debut and continue annually throughout the lifespan.[38] For female recipients of solid-organ transplants, cervical cancer screening should be performed annually post-transplant.[39] For women with abnormal screening tests, colposcopy with biopsy remains the current gold standard for diagnosing HPV-associated cervical lesions and invasive cancers in women who are immunocompetent and immunocompromised. Biopsies for histologic diagnosis of the cervix are directed to cervical changes noted by colposcopy.

Multiple U.S. Food and Drug Administration (FDA)–approved high-risk HPV tests are available for clinical use, including QIAGEN Hybrid Capture 2 (QIAGEN, Inc, Valencia, CA, USA) and the Cervista HPV HR high-risk screening test (Hologic, Inc, Madison, WI, USA). The FDA-approved indications for the use of these tests are (1) as adjunct screening for women aged 30 years or older, (2) for triage of ASCUS (atypical squamous cells of undetermined significance) cytology in women aged 21 years and older, and (3) in select follow-up situations after a diagnosis of high-grade CIN.[40] The tests are not recommended for: screening partners; screening men; testing women younger than 21 years; screening before HPV vaccination; or, diagnosing genital warts. No clinical indications exist regarding screening for low-risk HPV types.[32]

Currently no national recommendations exist regarding routine screening for anal cancer, partly because of the lack of consensus on the optimal method and frequency for screening. Some clinical centers with the capacity to evaluate screening perform anal cytology to screen high-risk populations for anal cancer.[41] In these centers, anal cytology is followed by HRA for those with abnormal cytologic results (eg, ASCUS or worse). HRA is performed in a manner similar to cervical colposcopy, with histology as the gold standard for diagnosing HPV-related AIN and cancer. For centers that are not performing cytology/HRA, an annual digital anal examination can be performed to detect masses on palpation that could be anal cancer. High-risk HPV tests are not clinically useful for anal cancer screening among MSM, because of a very high prevalence of anal HPV infection.[32] No published studies have described or compared the efficacy of various available screening methods for the prevention and/or early detection of anal cancer.

CLINICAL MANAGEMENT AND TREATMENT

Treatment is directed to the clinical manifestations of HPV infection, but not the infection itself. The treatment options differ depending on the condition/disease. Treatments for anogenital warts include patient-applied and provider administered therapies. Some patients elect to wait to see if genital warts regress on their own. Patients with warts that are located on the rectum or cervix, patients with extensive genital warts, and patients whose anogenital warts do not respond to a standard course of therapy should be managed by a specialist.

Table 2 describes recommended patient-applied and provider-administered therapies for genital warts, including recommended dosage and duration of therapy.[32] Patient-applied therapies include Podofilox 0.5% solution or gel, imiquimod 3.75% and 5% cream, and sinecatechins 15% ointment. Patient-applied therapies should only be used when the warts can be identified and accessed for treatment, and in patients with a high likelihood of compliance. A follow-up appointment several weeks into therapy to determine appropriateness of medication use and response to treatment may be useful. Provider-administered therapies include cryotherapy with liquid nitrogen or cryoprobe, trichloroacetic acid (TCA), or bichloroacetic acid 80% to 90%, and surgical removal. Other provider-administered therapies are also available, but with fewer data available and/or more reported side effects. Anogenital warts may be surgically removed through tangential scissor excision, tangential shave excision, curettage, electrosurgery, or other methods.

Recent changes to guidelines for the management of cervical squamous intraepithelial lesions recommend that CIN 1 be managed through follow-up rather than treatment, because these lesions often regress and the harms outweigh the benefits.[40]

Table 2
Recommended treatments for anogenital warts

External Anogenital Warts	Recommended Treatments	Dose/Route	Alternative Treatments
Patient-applied	Imiquimod 3.75%, 5% cream	Topically qhs 3× wk (5%) or qhs (3.75%) up to 16 wk	Intralesional interferon
	Podofilox 0.5% solution or gel	Topically bid × 3 d followed by 4 d no treatment for up to 4 cycles	Laser surgery Photodynamic therapy Topical cidofovir Podophyllin resin 10%–25%
	Sinecatechins 15% ointment	Topically tid for up to 16 wk	
Provider-applied	Cryotherapy	Apply once q1–2 wk	
	Bichloroacetic or trichloroacetic acid 80%–90%	Apply once q1–2 wk	
	Surgical removal		

Abbreviations: bid, twice a day; qhs, each evening; tid, three times a day; wk, week.
Data from Centers for Disease Control and Prevention. Sexually Transmitted Diseases Treatment Guidelines, 2010. MMWR Recomm Rep 2010;59(RR12):1–110; and Kim Workowski, personal communication, 2013.

Treatments for CIN 2 or 3 are tailored to the patient and may include the loop electrosurgical excision procedure, conization, laser, or cryotherapy. Treatment for adenocarcinoma in situ is generally either conization or hysterectomy. Treatments for cervical cancer depend on the stage of the cancer, size of the tumor, desire to preserve fertility, and patient age, and may include chemotherapy, radiation therapy, surgery, or other therapies.

Data are limited on the optimal treatments for high-grade AIN. Patient-applied modalities include intra-anal imiquimod and 5-fluorouracil. Provider-administered modalities include infrared coagulation, TCA, electrocautery, and surgical therapy, which is usually reserved for patients with extensive disease. Depending on treatment modality, per-lesion cure rates range from 63% to 85% after initial treatment based on retrospective studies,[42–44] but recurrence rates are high and range from 25% to 75% at 6 months to 1 year in HIV-infected MSM, and are similar (although slightly lower) in HIV-negative MSM.[42,43,45] No data show the impact of high-grade AIN treatment on prevention of incident anal cancer or cancer-related morbidity and mortality.

Anal cancer treatment varies according to stage and tumor location, and may include local excision alone, or excision with combined modality therapy composed of radiation and chemotherapy; in some cases, radical surgical therapy such as abdominoperineal resection is required.[46]

PREVENTION AND CONTROL

Two HPV vaccines are licensed for use in the United States. Quadrivalent HPV vaccine (Gardasil, Merck and Co, Inc, Whitehouse Station, NJ, USA) is licensed for use in women and men aged 9 through 26 years. Bivalent HPV vaccine (Cervarix, GlaxoSmithKline, Brentford, Middlesex, UK) is licensed for use in women aged 9 through 25 years. Both vaccines are virus-like particle vaccines and are made with the L1 major capsid protein of HPV. Neither vaccine is infectious, and neither contains thimerosal (mercury) or antibiotics.

Routine vaccination of 11- or 12-year-old boys and girls is recommended. Either vaccine is recommended for routine use in 11- or 12-year-old girls, and vaccination is recommended for 13- through 26-year-old women who have not received any or all of the vaccine doses.[47,48] Quadrivalent vaccine is recommended for routine use in 11- or 12-year-old boys, and vaccination is recommended for 13- through 21-year-old men who have not received any or all of the vaccine doses.[49] MSM should receive the vaccine through age 26 years.[49] Men and women with HIV infection (and other immunocompromised populations) should also receive the vaccine through age 26 years (**Table 3**).

Both vaccines have shown very high efficacy for preventing type-specific cervical precancers. Clinical trials of bivalent and quadrivalent HPV vaccine showed greater than 93% efficacy for preventing CIN 2, CIN 3, and AIS.[50,51] Quadrivalent HPV vaccine showed very high efficacy for preventing vaginal/vulvar precancers, anal precancers, and anogenital warts.[52–54]

Vaccination produces antibody titers higher than those after natural infection.[55] Among men and women aged 16 to 23 years, anti-HPV 6, 11, 16, and 18 geometric mean titers 1 month after the third dose of vaccine were higher than those observed in participants who were HPV-seropositive and polymerase chain reaction–negative at enrollment in the placebo group.[55] Studies have shown high antibody titers to vaccine types through 8 years,[56] and others are continuing to follow cohorts of vaccinated girls and boys to monitor long-term efficacy and immunogenicity.

Prelicensure and postlicensure safety evaluations of HPV vaccines have demonstrated an acceptable safety profile.[57] Prelicensure safety evaluations of vaccines found that the most common adverse effects were local, including pain at injection site, swelling, and erythema.[57] More than 56 million doses of quadrivalent HPV vaccine have been distributed in the United States.[57] Ongoing postlicensure safety evaluations have shown that among more than 20,000 reports in women after quadrivalent vaccine administration, 92.1% were classified as "nonserious"; the most commonly reported local symptoms were injection site pain, redness, and swelling.[57]

The vaccines are prophylactic, and have the highest efficacy when given before exposure to HPV infection (ie, before sexual debut). The vaccines do not have any therapeutic effect; clinical trials showed no efficacy on existing infection or disease.[58] Vaccination is routinely recommended for 11- or 12-year-old girls and boys to provide prevention before exposure to HPV.[47–49]

The National Immunization Survey-Teenagers has collected vaccination information for adolescents aged 13 to 17 years. In 2012, only 53.8% of girls had received more than 1 dose of HPV vaccine and only 33.4% had received all 3 doses of the series.[55] Despite the availability of safe and effective vaccines, HPV vaccination uptake among adolescent girls did not increase between 2011 and 2012.[57] Despite suboptimal uptake of the HPV vaccines in the United States, recent studies have shown its effect on reductions of HPV type-specific infection[59] and genital warts.[60,61]

Consistent and correct condom use may reduce the risk for HPV and HPV-associated diseases (eg, genital warts, cervical cancer). A limited number of prospective studies have been conducted on condom use and HPV; one prospective study among newly sexually active college women showed a 70% reduction in HPV infection when their partners used condoms consistently and correctly.[62] Abstaining from sexual activity (ie, refraining from any genital contact with another person) is the only way to prevent genital HPV infection. Sexually active men and women can lower their chances of getting HPV by limiting numbers of sex partners, or choosing a partner who has had no or few prior sex partners. Counseling messages about HPV may be useful to patients, and are included in **Box 1**.

Table 3
Advisory Committee on Immunization Practices HPV vaccine recommendations

	General Population Women	General Population Men	Immunocompromised Women	Immunocompromised Men[a]	Men Who Have Sex With Men
Vaccine	Either HPV 2, HPV 4	HPV 4	Either HPV 2, HPV 4	HPV 4	HPV 4
Recommendations	Routine at 11 or 12 y Vaccination through age 26 y	Routine at 11 or 12 y Vaccination through age 21 y	Routine at 11 or 12 y Vaccination through age 26 y	Routine at 11 or 12 y Vaccination through age 26 y	Routine at 11 or 12 y Vaccination through age 26 y

[a] Includes those with HIV infection, post transplant.
Abbreviations: HPV 2, bivalent HPV vaccine; HPV 4, quadrivalent HPV vaccine.
Data from Refs.[47–49]

Box 1
Key counseling messages for providers to offer patients

Epidemiology

- Most sexually active people will get HPV at some point.
- The types of HPV that cause genital warts are different from the types that can cause cancer.
- Most patients who acquire HPV will not have any disease.
- In persons with an intact immune system, most (90%) of HPV infections resolve within 2 years. HIV infection decreases the immune system's ability to clear HPV infection.

Transmission

- HPV is passed frequently between sex partners.
- HPV may be passed through vaginal or anal sex, other genital contact, and through oral sex.
- In rare cases, vertical transmission can occur from mother to child.
- Most often it is impossible to know which partner transmitted HPV to the other.
- Presence of HPV infection is not evidence of infidelity.
- Anogenital warts can develop months to years after acquiring HPV.
- HPV types causing anogenital warts can be transmitted even when there are no visible signs of warts.

Genital warts

- If left untreated, genital warts may go away, stay the same, or increase in size or number.
- Genital warts do not typically develop into cancer; however, a patient with warts can have coexisting precancer, and this may be more likely in patients who are immunocompromised (eg, HIV-infected).
- Women with genital warts do not need more frequent Papanicolaou tests than other women.

Genital wart treatment

- Recurrences are common, especially in the first 3 months after treatment.
- Two types of treatments are available: patient-applied and provider-administered.

Partner management and disclosure

- Patients with a current diagnosis of warts should inform their partners because of risk of transmission.
- It is unclear whether informing future partners about a past diagnosis of genital warts will provide any health benefit to the partner.
- Partners may benefit from being tested for other sexually transmitted infections and HIV.
- Patients with active warts should avoid sexual activity with new partners until the warts are gone or removed. However, HPV may remain and be transmitted to partners even after visible warts are gone.

Prevention

- Effective HPV vaccines are available and recommended routinely for 11- or 12-year-old boys and girls.
- Two vaccines (Cervarix and Gardasil) protect against most cases of cervical cancer, and one vaccine (Gardasil) protects against genital warts and has been shown to protect against anal, vaginal and vulvar cancers. These vaccines are given in 3 doses over 6 months. Vaccines are most effective when all doses are received well before any sexual activity.

- Vaccines are also recommended through age 21 years for men (immunocompromised, HIV-infected, and MSM should receive them through age 26 years), and through age 26 years for women.
- Condoms may lower the risk of acquiring HPV; however, they are not fully protective.
- Abstinence and limiting the number of sex partners may decrease the risk of HPV acquisition/transmission.

REFERENCES

1. Satterwhite CW, Torrone E, Meites E, et al. Sexually transmitted infections among US women and men: prevalence and incidence estimates, 2008. Sex Transm Dis 2013;40(3):187–93.
2. Chesson HW, Ekwueme DU, Saraiya M, et al. The cost-effectiveness of male HPV vaccination in the United States. Vaccine 2012;30:6016–9.
3. Patel H, Wagner M, Singhal P, et al. Systematic review of the incidence and prevalence of genital warts. BMC Infect Dis 2013;13:39.
4. Hoy T, Singhal PK, Willey VJ, et al. Assessing incidence and economic burden of genital warts with data from a US commercially insured population. Curr Med Res Opin 2009;10:2343–51.
5. Insinga RP, Dasbach EJ, Myers ER. The health and economic burden of genital warts in a set of private health plans in the United States. Clin Infect Dis 2003;36:1397–403.
6. Koshiol JE, Laurent SA, Pimenta JM. Rate and predictors of new genital warts claims and genital warts–related healthcare utilization among privately insured patients in the United States. Sex Transm Dis 2004;31:748–52.
7. Armstrong LR, Preston EJ, Reichert M, et al. Incidence and prevalence of recurrent respiratory papillomatosis among children in Atlanta and Seattle. Clin Infect Dis 2000;31:107–9.
8. Jemal A, Simard EP, Dorell C. Annual Report to the Nation on the Status of Cancer, 1975-2009, featuring the burden and trends in human papillomavirus (HPV)-associated cancers and HPV vaccination coverage levels. J Natl Cancer Inst 2013;105(3):175–201.
9. Gillison ML, Chaturvedi AK, Lowy DR. HPV prophylactic vaccines and the potential prevention of noncervical cancers in both men and women. Cancer 2008;113:3036–46.
10. Silverberg MJ, Lau B, Justice AC, et al. Risk of anal cancer in HIV-infected and HIV-uninfected individuals in North America. Clin Infect Dis 2012;54(7):1026–34.
11. Piketty C, Selinger-Leneman H, Bouvier AM, et al. Incidence of HIV-related anal cancer remains increased despite long-term combined antiretroviral treatment: results from the French hospital database on HIV. Clin Oncol 2012;30:4360–6.
12. Dolev JC, Maurer T, Springer G, et al. Incidence and risk factors for verrucae in women. AIDS 2008;19:1213–9.
13. Winer RL, Lee SK, Hughes JP, et al. Genital human papillomavirus infection: incidence and risk factors in a cohort of female university students. Am J Epidemiol 2003;157:218–26.
14. Winer RL, Feng Q, Hughes JP, et al. Risk of female human papillomavirus acquisition associated with first male sex partner. J Infect Dis 2008;197(2):279–82.

15. Ho GY, Bierman R, Beardsley L, et al. Natural history of cervicovaginal papillomavirus infection in young women. N Engl J Med 1998;338(7):423–8.

16. Moscicki AB, Shiboski S, Broering J, et al. The natural history of human papillomavirus infection as measured by repeated DNA testing in adolescent and young women. J Pediatr 1998;132(2):277–84.

17. Giuliano AR, Lee JH, Fulp W, et al. Incidence and clearance of genital human papillomavirus infection in men (HIM): a cohort study. Lancet 2011;377: 932–40.

18. Hariri S, Unger ER, Sternberg M, et al. Prevalence of genital human papillomavirus among females in the United States, the National Health And Nutrition Examination Survey, 2003-2006. J Infect Dis 2011;204:566–73.

19. Chin-Hong PV, Vittinghoff E, Cranston RD, et al. Age-Specific prevalence of anal human papillomavirus infection in HIV-negative sexually active men who have sex with men: the EXPLORE study. J Infect Dis 2004;190(12):2070–6.

20. Giuliano AR, Lu B, Nielson CM, et al. Age-specific prevalence, incidence, and duration of human papillomavirus infections in a cohort of 290 US men. J Infect Dis 2008;198:827–35.

21. Shew ML, Weaver B, Tu W, et al. High frequency of human papillomavirus detection in the vagina before first vaginal intercourse among females enrolled in a longitudinal cohort study. J Infect Dis 2013;207:1012–5.

22. Marrazzo JM, Gorgos L. Emerging sexual health issues among women who have sex with women. Curr Infect Dis Rep, in press.

23. Burchell AN, Coutlée F, Tellier PP, et al. Genital transmission of human papillomavirus in recently formed heterosexual couples. J Infect Dis 2011;204(11): 1723–9.

24. Hernandez BY, Wilkens LR, Zhu X, et al. Transmission of human papillomavirus in heterosexual couples. Emerg Infect Dis 2008;14(6):888–94.

25. Widdice L, Ma Y, Jonte J, et al. Concordance and transmission of human papillomavirus within heterosexual couples observed over short intervals. J Infect Dis 2013;207(8):1286–94.

26. Reiter PL, Pendergraft WF 3rd, Brewer NT. Meta-analysis of human papillomavirus infection concordance. Cancer Epidemiol Biomarkers Prev 2010;19(11): 2916–31.

27. Anic GM, Lee JH, Stockwell H, et al. Incidence and human papillomavirus (HPV) type distribution of genital warts in a multinational cohort of men: the HPV in men study. J Infect Dis 2011;204(12):1886–92.

28. Arima Y, Winer RL, Feng Q, et al. Development of genital warts after incident detection of human papillomavirus infection in young men. J Infect Dis 2010; 202(8):1181–4.

29. Garland SM, Steben M, Sings HL, et al. Natural history of genital warts: analysis of the placebo arm of 2 randomized phase iii trials of a quadrivalent human papillomavirus (types 6, 11, 16, and 18) vaccine. J Infect Dis 2009;199:805–14.

30. Winer RL, Kiviat NB, Hughes JP, et al. Development and duration of human papillomavirus lesions after initial infection. J Infect Dis 2005;191(5):731–8.

31. Woodhall SC, Jit M, Cai C, et al. Cost of treatment and QALYs lost due to genital warts: data for the economic evaluation of HPV vaccines in the United Kingdom. Sex Transm Dis 2009;36:515–21.

32. Centers for Disease Control and Prevention. Sexually transmitted diseases treatment guidelines, 2010. MMWR Recomm Rep 2010;59(RR12):1–110.

33. Ostor AG. Natural history of cervical intraepithelial neoplasia: a critical review. Int J Gynecol Pathol 1993;12(2):186–92.

34. Castle PE, Schiffman M, Wheeler CM, et al. Evidence for frequent regression of cervical intraepithelial neoplasia-grade 2. Obstet Gynecol 2009;113(1):18–25.

35. Edge SB, Byrd DR, Compton CC, et al, editors. AJCC cancer staging manual. 7th edition. New York: Springer; 2010. p. 165–73.

36. Hoots BE, Palefsky JM, Pimenta JM, et al. Human papillomavirus type distribution in anal cancer and anal intraepithelial lesions. Int J Cancer 2009;124(10): 2375–83.

37. Centers for Disease Control and Prevention-Division of Cancer Prevention and Control. Cervical Cancer Screening Guidelines for Average-Risk Women. Available at: http://www.cdc.gov/cancer/cervical/pdf/guidelines.pdf. Accessed August 3, 2012.

38. Panel on Opportunistic Infections in HIV-Infected Adults and Adolescents. Guidelines for the prevention and treatment of opportunistic infections in HIV-infected adults and adolescents: recommendations from the Centers for Disease Control and Prevention, the National Institutes of Health, and the HIV Medicine Association of the Infectious Diseases Society of America. Available at: http://aidsinfo.nih.gov/contentfiles/lvguidelines/adult_oi.pdf. Accessed August 3, 2013.

39. Kidney Disease, Improving Global Outcomes (KDIGO) Transplant Work Group. KDIGO clinical practice guideline for the care of kidney transplant recipients. Am J Transplant 2009;9(Suppl 3):S1–155.

40. Massad LS, Einstein MH, Huh WK, et al. 2012 ASCCP Consensus Guidelines Conference. 2012 updated consensus guidelines for the management of abnormal cervical cancer screening tests and cancer precursors. Obstet Gynecol 2013;121(4):829–46.

41. University of California San Francisco, Anal Cancer Info: HRA Providers. Available at: http://id.medicine.ucsf.edu/analcancerinfo/providers.html. Accessed October 10, 2013.

42. Goldstone RN, Goldstone AB, Russ J, et al. Long-term follow-up of infrared coagulator ablation of anal high-grade dysplasia in men who have sex with men. Dis Colon Rectum 2011;54(10):1284–92.

43. Marks DK, Goldstone SE. Electrocautery ablation of high-grade anal squamous intraepithelial lesions in HIV-negative and HIV-positive men who have sex with men. J Acquir Immune Defic Syndr 2012;59(3):259–65.

44. Nathan M, Hickey N, Mayuranathan L, et al. Treatment of anal human papillomavirus-associated disease: a long term outcome study. Int J STD AIDS 2008;19(7):445–9.

45. Singh JC, Kuohung V, Palefsky JM. Efficacy of trichloroacetic acid in the treatment of anal intraepithelial neoplasia in HIV-positive and HIV-negative men who have sex with men [Erratum in J Acquir Immune Defic Syndr 2012;60(3):e105–6]. J Acquir Immune Defic Syndr 2009;52(4):474–9.

46. National Cancer Institute: PDQ Anal Cancer Treatment. Bethesda (MD): National Cancer Institute. Available at: http://cancer.gov/cancertopics/pdq/treatment/anal/HealthProfessional. Accessed October 10, 2013.

47. Markowitz LE, Dunne EF, Saraiya M, et al. Quadrivalent human papillomavirus vaccine: recommendations of the Advisory Committee on Immunization Practices (ACIP). MMWR Recomm Rep 2007;56(RR-2):1–24.

48. Centers for Disease Control and Prevention. FDA Licensure of Bivalent Human Papillomavirus Vaccine (HPV2, Cervarix) for Use in Females and Updated HPV Vaccination Recommendations from the Advisory Committee on Immunization Practices (ACIP). MMWR Recomm Rep 2010;59:626–9.

49. Centers for Disease Control and Prevention. Recommendations on the use of quadrivalent human papillomavirus vaccine in males—Advisory Committee on Immunization Practices (ACIP), 2011. MMWR Morb Mortal Wkly Rep 2011;60: 1705–8.

50. Paavonen J, Naud P, Salmerón J, et al. Efficacy of human papillomavirus (HPV)-16/18 AS04-adjuvanted vaccine against cervical infection and precancer caused by oncogenic HPV types (Patricia): final analysis of a double-blind, randomized study in young women. Lancet 2009;374:301–14.

51. Kjaer SK, Sigurdsson K, Iversen OE, et al. A Pooled analysis of continued prophylactic efficacy of quadrivalent human papillomavirus (Types 6/11/16/18) vaccine against high-grade cervical and external genital lesions. Cancer Prev Res (Phila) 2009;2(10):868–77.

52. Joura EA, Leodolter S, Hernandez-Avila M, et al. Efficacy of a quadrivalent prophylactic human papillomavirus (types 6, 11, 16, 18) L1 virus-like-particle vaccine against high-grade vulval and vaginal lesions: a combined analysis of three randomized clinical trials. Lancet 2007;369:1693–702.

53. Palefsky JM, Giuliano AR, Goldstone S, et al. HPV Vaccine against Anal HPV Infection and Anal Intraepithelial Neoplasia. N Engl J Med 2011;365:1576–85.

54. FUTURE I/II Study Group. Four year efficacy of prophylactic human papillomavirus quadrivalent vaccine against low grade cervical, vulvar, and vaginal intraepithelial neoplasia and anogenital warts: randomized controlled trial. BMJ 2010;340:1–9.

55. Schiller JT, Castellsague X, Garland SM. A review of clinical trials of human papillomavirus prophylactic vaccines. Vaccine 2012;30:123–38.

56. Roteli-Martins C, Naud P, De Borba P, et al. Sustained immunogenicity and efficacy of the HPV-16/18 AS04-adjuvanted vaccine: up to 8.4 years of follow-up. Hum Vaccin Immunother 2012;8(3):390–7.

57. Centers for Disease Control and Prevention (CDC). Human papillomavirus vaccination coverage among adolescent girls, 2007-2012, and postlicensure vaccine safety monitoring, 2006-2013-United States. MMWR Morb Mortal Wkly Rep 2013;62(29):591–5.

58. Hildasheim A, Herrero R, Wacholder S, et al. Effect of human papillomavirus 16/18 L1 viruslike particle vaccine among young women with preexisting infection: a randomized trial. JAMA 2007;298(7):743–53.

59. Markowitz LE, Hariri S, Lin C, et al. Reduction in human papillomavirus (HPV) prevalence among young women following HPV vaccine introduction in the United States, National Health and Nutrition Examination Surveys, 2003-2010. J Infect Dis 2013;208(3):385–93.

60. Flagg EW, Schwartz R, Weinstock H. Prevalence of anogenital warts among participants in private health plans in the United States, 2003-2010: potential impact of human papillomavirus vaccination. Am J Public Health 2013;103(8): 1428–35.

61. Bauer HM, Wright G, Chow J. Evidence of human papillomavirus vaccine effectiveness in reducing genital warts: an analysis of California public family planning administrative claims data, 2007-2010. Am J Public Health 2012;102(5): 833–5.

62. Winer RL, Hughes JP, Feng Q, et al. Condom use and the risk of genital human papillomavirus infection in young women. N Engl J Med 2006;354(25):2645–54.

Mycoplasma genitalium
An Emergent Sexually Transmitted Disease?

Lisa E. Manhart, PhD[a,b],*

KEYWORDS

- *Mycoplasma genitalium* • Urethritis • NGU • Cervicitis • Pelvic inflammatory disease
- STD • STI

KEY POINTS

- *Mycoplasma genitalium* is found in 1% to 3% of the general population, less commonly than *Chlamydia trachomatis* but more commonly than *Neisseria gonorrhoeae.*
- Strong and consistent evidence indicates that *M genitalium* causes nongonococcal urethritis in men.
- Building evidence links *M genitalium* with cervicitis, pelvic inflammatory disease, and infertility in women.
- Individuals infected with *M genitalium* have twice the risk of human immunodeficiency virus (HIV) infection and may be more likely to transmit HIV in cases of dual infection.
- Standard therapies for male and female genital tract syndromes have poor efficacy against *M genitalium*, although moxifloxacin has been effective for treatment failures.

INTRODUCTION

The last newly recognized sexually transmitted infection was identified more than 40 years ago when *Chlamydia trachomatis* was recognized as a genital tract pathogen in the early 1970s.[1] Since that time, no new sexually transmitted pathogens have been definitively determined, although *Mycoplasma genitalium* has been considered an emerging sexually transmitted disease (STD) for several years. *M genitalium* was first identified in 1980[2] and epidemiologic studies of its association with STD syndromes have been conducted since the development of nucleic acid amplification assays in the early 1990s.[3,4] An increasing body of literature describes studies of the association of this bacterium with reproductive tract infections, including nongonococcal urethritis (NGU) in men and cervicitis, endometritis, pelvic inflammatory disease (PID), infertility, and adverse birth outcomes in women. As the evidence grows, consistent trends are

Conflict of Interest: L.E. Manhart previously received study drugs from Pfizer, Inc and diagnostic test reagents from Gen-Probe, Inc.
a Department of Epidemiology, University of Washington, Seattle, WA, USA; b Department of Global Health, University of Washington, Seattle, WA, USA
* UW Center for AIDS and STD, 325 9th Avenue, Seattle, WA 98104.
E-mail address: lmanhart@u.washington.edu

becoming evident, suggesting that *M genitalium* is no longer an emerging STD, but that it now merits the definition of what is classically defined as an STD.

M GENITALIUM: THE BACTERIUM

M genitalium is a bacterium of the Mollicutes class, characterized by the absence of a cell wall. As a result it is not detectable by Gram staining, and is not susceptible to cell wall synthesis–inhibiting antimicrobials such as penicillins, cephalosporins, or poly-peptide/antimycobacterial antibiotics. *M genitalium* is among the smallest known bacteria,[5] making it the target of efforts to determine the minimal requirements for life[6] and to create the first chemically synthesized bacterium.[7] It possesses a characteristic flask shape (**Fig. 1**) and, perhaps because of its small size, is fastidious. Culture is time consuming and difficult, requires cocultivation in Vero cells,[8] and can take up to several months to show growth. Only a few laboratories in the world have accomplished this feat; therefore, culture cannot be considered the gold standard, nor is it a useful tool for clinical detection. However, very sensitive and specific nucleic acid amplification tests in the form of polymerase chain reaction (PCR) and transcription-mediated amplification assays have been developed. With the use of these assays, *M genitalium* has been detected in the male urethra, rectum, and epididymis. Male circumcision has been associated with a nearly 50% reduction in risk for *M genitalium*[9] (unlike *C trachomatis*, *Neisseria gonorrhoeae*, and *Trichomonas vaginalis*[10]), suggesting that the foreskin may be an additional site of colonization. *M genitalium* has also been detected in the female vagina, cervix, endometrium, and fallopian tubes, and a growing body of literature has examined its relationship with both male and female reproductive tract disease syndromes.[11]

M GENITALIUM: EPIDEMIOLOGY

The prevalence of *M genitalium* in general population samples ranges from 1% to 3%[12–14]; lower than the prevalence of *C trachomatis*, but higher than the prevalence of *N gonorrhoeae*. In higher risk populations, such as STD clinic attendees and individuals with compatible clinical syndromes, the prevalence is higher, ranging from 2% to 33%.

M genitalium was first identified in 2 of 13 urethral specimens from men with NGU[2]; so early studies were focused on determining whether the bacterium caused male

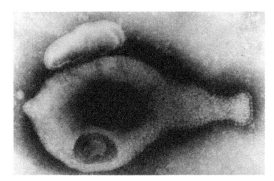

Fig. 1. Transmission electron micrograph of *M genitalium*. (*From* Tully JG, Taylor-Robinson D, Rose DL, et al. *Mycoplasma genitalium*, a new species from the human urogenital tract. Int J Syst Bacteriol 1983;33:391; with permission.)

urethritis. Since the initial discovery, a total of 33 studies in high-income countries have evaluated the association between *M genitalium* and male urethritis, nearly all of which reported significant associations with NGU, with odds ratios (ORs) ranging from 3.2 to 20.3 (**Table 1**).[15–47] *M genitalium* is found in approximately 15% (range, 5%–33%) of men with NGU, and in approximately 22% of men with nonchlamydial NGU. Despite being more strongly associated with NGU in the absence than in the presence of *C trachomatis*, *C trachomatis*/*M genitalium* coinfections are common in some settings, and clinical characteristics of men infected with *M genitalium* resemble those of men infected with *C trachomatis* more so than those of men infected with *N gonorrhoeae*.[33] Nevertheless, *M genitalium* infections are not characterized by a unique clinical syndrome,[48] making it difficult to identify *M genitalium* infections from clinical signs or symptoms.

Depending on the setting, *M genitalium* can account for a large proportion of persistent and/or recurrent cases of NGU. In a recent clinical trial, *M genitalium* was the most prevalent of all identified causes in men who experienced clinical treatment failure; 33% of men with persisting signs and symptoms of NGU had *M genitalium*, compared with only 9% with *C trachomatis* and 12% with *T vaginalis*.[49] In other studies, the prevalence of *M genitalium* among men with persistent or recurrent NGU has ranged from 13% to 41%,[23,50–53] with the highest prevalence among men who were originally treated with a doxycycline regimen[51] (discussed later).

M genitalium has been detected in the epididymis and the rectum, but at low prevalence (2%–9% in men with epididymitis[54–56] and 1.6%–11% in the rectum in studies of men who have sex with men [MSM][43,57–60]). No studies have compared men with

Table 1
Associations with and prevalence of *M genitalium* in sexually transmitted infection (STI) syndromes

STI Syndrome	Association with *M genitalium*; Strength of Evidence	Prevalence in Persons with the Syndrome[a] (%)
Acute nongonococcal urethritis	Strong; evidence suggests a causal relationship	5–33
Persistent nongonococcal urethritis	Strong; evidence suggests a causal relationship	13–41
Epididymitis	Poor; limited evidence	2–9
Proctitis	Poor; limited evidence	12
Cervicitis	Moderate; evidence is conflicting but suggests an association	2–29
PID	Moderate to strong; most evidence supports a causal relationship, but some is conflicting	4–18 17–39[b]
Infertility	Moderate; evidence is conflicting but suggests an association	20 17–22[b]
Preterm birth	Modest; evidence is conflicting and is of modest quality	0–8
Ectopic pregnancy	Poor; limited evidence	18[b]
Human immunodeficiency virus infection	Strong; evidence suggests a causal relationship	2–33

[a] Nucleic acid amplification test detection in urine, swab, or tissue specimens, unless otherwise specified.
[b] Serologic detection of antibodies to *M genitalium*.

and without epididymitis, and 3 of the 4 studies evaluating rectal carriage reported no significant association of *M genitalium* with rectal symptoms or proctitis.[43,57–59] Taken together, the available evidence suggests that *M genitalium* does not play a large role in these syndromes. However, rectal carriage may serve as a reservoir for transmission in MSM, resulting in urethral infection and potentially NGU in male partners.

Cervicitis has been referred to as the female counterpart of male urethritis,[61] and therefore it might be hypothesized that associations with *M genitalium* and cervicitis would mirror those with urethritis in men. Although more than half (60%) of the 15 studies in high-income countries[15,62–75] showed significant associations with cervicitis,[15,62,65,66,70–73,75] this relationship is not as strong as the associations for male syndromes, with ORs between 1.2 and 5.7. In general, studies that did not show a significant association between *M genitalium* and cervicitis[68,69,76] relied on chart review and abstraction of clinical diagnoses, whereas studies that defined cervicitis as objective evidence of cervical inflammation ($\geq$30 polymorphonuclear leukocytes per high-power field) did show an association,[15,64,67,70,71,73] although not always statistically significant.[64,67,73] *M genitalium* is found in approximately 10% (range, 2%–29%) of women with cervicitis. Thus, available evidence suggests a causal association between *M genitalium* and objectively defined cervicitis. Similar to the epidemiology of NGU in men, chlamydial coinfections are common in some settings.[66,68,77] The clinical manifestations of endocervical *M genitalium* infection resemble chlamydial more than gonococcal infections[65] (eg, less profuse mucopus at the cervical os). Although few studies have reported associations with *M genitalium* and vaginal inflammation or vaginal discharge,[71,78] several have reported associations with dysuria and urethritis in women, with ORs from studies in Western settings ranging from 2.1 to 3.4,[15,67,73] suggesting that *M genitalium* can infect the female urethra.

PID is a polymicrobial syndrome[79] often characterized by anaerobic bacterial species,[80] and *M genitalium* is a facultative anaerobe. Results from early serologic studies of *M genitalium*'s contribution to the multiple causes of PID were mixed,[81–83] possibly because of cross reactivity of the serum antibody assays with *Mycoplasma pneumoniae*. In contrast, when nucleic acid amplification tests have been used to detect *M genitalium* in the female reproductive tract, studies have consistently reported increased risk of endometritis[84–88] and/or clinically diagnosed PID[62,89–93] in the presence of this organism. Postabortal PID has been less frequently studied, but was strongly associated with *M genitalium* (adjusted OR [AOR], 6.3; 1.6–25.3) in a study of Swedish women.[91] The organism has also been detected in the fallopian tube of a woman with mild salpingitis, showing its ability to ascend in the upper reproductive tract,[91] and studies in nonhuman primates in which endosalpingitis was induced after inoculation with *M genitalium*[94] suggest a causal role in PID. Clinical characteristics of *M genitalium*–associated PID seem to be more similar to those of women with chlamydial than gonococcal PID,[88,95] but the frequency with which women infected with *M genitalium* experience PID remains unknown.

Studies of *M genitalium* and infertility, adverse birth outcomes, and ectopic pregnancy have been hampered by a low prevalence of *M genitalium* in the populations studied. Although this may reflect the low-risk nature of the populations studied, it also suggests that, if *M genitalium* does play a role in these disease syndromes, it probably only accounts for a small proportion of cases. Only 1 study has evaluated the association of *M genitalium* with ectopic pregnancy.[83] In contrast, the strongest data suggest an association with infertility. Two Danish studies that accounted for prior infection with *C trachomatis* both observed a 4-fold higher likelihood of prior *M genitalium* infection among women with tubal factor infertility relative to other causes of infertility (AORs, 4.2–4.5).[96,97] Additionally, a study using PCR reported a

9-fold increased risk of idiopathic infertility among women with *M genitalium* detected in cervical swab specimens or peritoneal aspirate (OR, 9.1; 1.0–426; P = .05).[98] Among men, *M genitalium* has been detected in 2% to 5% of infertile men,[99,100] but there were no comparison groups of fertile men in these studies, so there is insufficient evidence to determine whether it is associated with male infertility.

Studies of the relationship between *M genitalium* and preterm delivery[101–107] have produced mixed results, partly because of the uncommon nature of premature birth in several of the prospective studies (2%–6%).[103,104] In these longitudinal assessments, *M genitalium* prevalence was also low (0.7%–0.8%) and each reported no association with preterm birth. However, a US-based study reported a 2.5-fold increased risk of preterm delivery in women with *M genitalium* who presented with uterine contractions at 23 to 32 weeks' gestation (AOR, 2.5; 1.2–6.0),[105] similar to results from a study in Peru (AOR, 2.5; 95% confidence interval, 1.2–5.0).[106] These data suggest that, when present, *M genitalium* may play a causal role in preterm delivery.

HUMAN IMMUNODEFICIENCY VIRUS INFECTION AND *M GENITALIUM*

According to a recent meta-analysis, individuals infected with *M genitalium* are twice as likely to be infected with human immunodeficiency virus (HIV) (summary OR, 2.0; 1.4–2.8),[108] and nearly all of the additional reports published since[43,78,109–117] have confirmed a strong association between *M genitalium* and HIV infection. All were either cross-sectional or retrospective reports; thus, the possibility of common risk behavior explaining this observation, without invoking a biologic interaction, could not be ruled out. However, 2 studies among African women showed that *M genitalium* infection preceded HIV infection, suggesting a potential role for *M genitalium* in the promotion of subsequent HIV-1 acquisition. In a nested case-control study in Zimbabwe and Uganda, risk of HIV acquisition was nearly 2.5 times more likely among women who had been diagnosed with *M genitalium* ~12 weeks earlier (AOR, 2.4; 1.01–5.80)[116] and high-risk women with an *M genitalium* infection at enrollment in a Ugandan study were twice as likely to subsequently test positive for HIV than *M genitalium*–negative women (adjusted hazard ratio, 2.2; 1.11–4.36).[117] In addition to increased risk for acquiring HIV, *M genitalium* may also increase shedding of HIV virus among dually infected persons, thereby increasing the risk of HIV transmission. Two of 3 studies reported that HIV-1 viral shedding was increased in persons infected with *M genitalium*,[109,114] although 1 study did not.[113]

TREATMENT

Despite the availability of assays to detect *M genitalium* in research settings, there is currently no diagnostic test approved by the US Food and Drug Administration (FDA) on the market in the United States. Therefore, most individuals infected with *M genitalium* receive one of the recommended syndromic therapies for NGU or cervicitis (doxycycline 100 mg twice a day × 7days or azithromycin 1 g single dose). Of these two regimens, azithromycin is the more effective. The median microbiologic cure rate for *M genitalium* after doxycycline is only 38% (**Table 2**). Azithromycin (1 g single dose) has been considered the preferred therapy for *M genitalium* infections, and early reports of microbiologic cure rates were high (82%–100%).[22,51,118,119] However, resistance to azithromycin has rapidly emerged, and microbiologic cure rates for the standard azithromycin regimen have declined dramatically. In 2 recent clinical trials, they were only 67%[120] and 40%.[121] Moxifloxacin (400 mg × 7–14 days) has been used to successfully treat cases of known *M genitalium* treatment failure, and cure rates have been excellent (100%).[122–129] However, treatment failures with the 7-day regimen

Table 2
Efficacy of standard STI treatment regimens against *M genitalium*

STI Syndrome	Treatment Regimen	Number of Studies	Microbiologic Cure: Median, Range (%)
Nongonococcal urethritis	Doxycycline[a]	11	38, 0–94
	Azithromycin 1 g single dose	14	84, 40–98
	Azithromycin extended dose[b]	7	93, 60–100
	Moxifloxacin[c]	6	100, 100–100
	Levofloxacin/ofloxacin[d]	3	44, 33–60
	Gatifloxacin[e]	2	92, 83–100
	Sitafloxacin[f]	1	100
Cervicitis	Doxycycline[a]	4	42, 29–100
	Azithromycin 1 g single dose	7	88, 79–96
	Azithromycin extended dose[b]	5	100, 78–100
	Moxifloxacin[c]	8	100, 91–100
	Levofloxacin/ofloxacin[d]	2	55, 44–71
	Sitafloxacin[f]	1	86, 79–92
PID	Moxifloxacin 400 mg × 14 d	1	100
	Ofloxacin 400 mg bid plus Metronidazole 500 mg bid × 14 d	1	100
	Cefoxitin 2 g parenterally every 6 h plus doxycycline 100 mg bid × 14 d (inpatient)	1[g]	57, 56–59
	Cefoxitin 2 g IM plus probenecid 1 g plus doxycycline 100 mg bid × 14 d (outpatient)	1[g]	57, 56–59

Abbreviations: bid, twice a day; IM, intramuscularly.
 [a] Doxycycline regimens: 200 mg plus 100 mg × 13 days; 200 mg plus 200 mg twice a day × 7 to 8 days; 100 mg × 7 days; 100 mg twice a day × 7 days.
 [b] Azithromycin extended-dose regimen: 500 mg on day 1 plus 250 mg × 4 days.
 [c] Moxifloxacin given for NGU and cervicitis treatment failures in all cases but 1 (Terada and colleagues,[125] 2012). Regimens include 400 mg × 7 to 14 days, all treatment failures occurred after the 7-day regimen.
 [d] Levofloxacin regimens: 100 mg 3 times a day × 14 days; 500 mg × 7 days; and 500 mg × 14 days. Ofloxacin regimen: 200 mg twice a day × 10 days.
 [e] Gatifloxacin regimen: 200 mg twice a day × 7 days.
 [f] Sitafloxacin regimens: 100 mg twice a day × 7 days; 200 mg × 7 days; 200 mg × 14 days.
 [g] Single study tested inpatient and outpatient PID regimens and reported cure rates for both regimens combined (*M genitalium* detected in endometrium/cervix and endometrium alone).

have recently been reported,[125] and moxifloxacin resistance may also be emerging. Older macrolides (levofloxacin and ofloxacin) are not considered effective against *M genitalium*, although newer macrolides not on the US market (gatifloxacin, sitaflox-acin) have microbiologic cure rates of 86% to 100%. Standard regimens for PID, which include antibiotics that inhibit cell wall synthesis paired with doxycycline, have a median failure rate of 57% and are not generally effective. However, moxiflox-acin and a combined regimen of ofloxacin and metronidazole were effective in a small group of women.[130]

FUTURE CHALLENGES

In the 30 years since its first identification, *M genitalium* has emerged as a sexually transmitted pathogen. Consistent evidence from well-designed epidemiologic studies has shown a strong association between *M genitalium* infection and male urethritis, and it is now widely recognized as a cause of NGU. Treatment failure is common and, in many settings, *M genitalium* is the most frequently detected pathogen among men with persistent NGU. Although the evidence for female STD syndromes is less consistent, it suggests that *M genitalium* is also associated with female reproductive tract syndromes (cervicitis, endometritis, PID) and likely with some of the adverse sequelae often related to these syndromes (tubal infertility and preterm birth). Future studies should focus on definitive evaluations of links between new *M genitalium* infections and incident female syndromes, with an emphasis on studies of the most severe sequelae (eg, infertility, ectopic pregnancy, and adverse birth outcomes). In recognizing *M genitalium* as an STD, 2 particular challenges to clinical care are evident: there is as yet no FDA-approved diagnostic test, and effective treatment options seem to be increasingly limited. New diagnostic assays are being developed but, in the interim, clinicians must rely on their clinical judgment to diagnose and treat *M genitalium* infections. *M genitalium* should be suspected in cases of persistent urethritis, cervicitis, and PID, and antimicrobial therapy should be adjusted accordingly. Given the waning efficacy of azithromycin in many settings, moxifloxacin therapy should be considered when *M genitalium* is suspected, and systems to monitor the prevalence of macrolide resistance should be developed to guide treatment decisions.

REFERENCES

1. Stamm WE. *Chlamydia trachomatis* infections of the adult. In: Holmes KK, Sparling PF, Stamm WE, et al, editors. Sexually transmitted diseases. 4th edition. New York: McGraw-Hill; 2008. p. 575–94.
2. Tully JG, Cole RM, Taylor-Robinson D, et al. A newly discovered *Mycoplasma* in the human urogenital tract. Lancet 1981;1(8233):1288–91.
3. Jensen JS, Uldum SA, Sondergard-Andersen J, et al. Polymerase chain reaction for detection of *Mycoplasma genitalium* in clinical samples. J Clin Microbiol 1991;29:46–50.
4. Palmer HM, Gilroy CB, Furr PM, et al. Development and evaluation of the polymerase chain reaction to detect *Mycoplasma genitalium*. FEMS Microbiol Lett 1991;61:199–203.
5. Fraser CM, Gocayne JD, White O, et al. The minimal gene complement of *Mycoplasma genitalium*. Science 1995;270:397–403.
6. Glass JI, Assad-Garcia N, Alperovich N, et al. Essential genes of a minimal bacterium. Proc Natl Acad Sci U S A 2006;103:425–30.
7. Gibson DG, Benders GA, Andrews-Pfannkoch C, et al. Complete chemical synthesis, assembly, and cloning of a *Mycoplasma genitalium* genome. Science 2008;319:1215–20.
8. Jensen JS, Hansen HT, Lind K. Isolation of *Mycoplasma genitalium* strains from the male urethra. J Clin Microbiol 1996;34:286–91.
9. Mehta SD, Gaydos C, Maclean I, et al. The effect of medical male circumcision on urogenital *Mycoplasma genitalium* among men in Kisumu, Kenya. Sex Transm Dis 2012;39:276–80.
10. Mehta SD, Moses S, Agot K, et al. Adult male circumcision does not reduce the risk of incident *Neisseria gonorrhoeae*, *Chlamydia trachomatis*, or *Trichomonas vaginalis* infection: results from a randomized, controlled trial in Kenya. J Infect Dis 2009;200:370–8.
11. Taylor-Robinson D, Jensen JS. *Mycoplasma genitalium*: from chrysalis to multicolored butterfly. Clin Microbiol Rev 2011;24:498–514.

12. Andersen B, Sokolowski I, Ostergaard L, et al. *Mycoplasma genitalium*: prevalence and behavioural risk factors in the general population. Sex Transm Infect 2007;83:237–41.
13. Manhart LE, Holmes KK, Hughes JP, et al. *Mycoplasma genitalium* among young adults in the United States: an emerging sexually transmitted infection. Am J Public Health 2007;97:1118–25.
14. Oakeshott P, Kerry S, Aghaizu A, et al. Randomised controlled trial of screening for *Chlamydia trachomatis* to prevent pelvic inflammatory disease: the POPI (prevention of pelvic infection) trial. BMJ 2010;340:c1642.
15. Anagrius C, Lore B, Jensen JS. *Mycoplasma genitalium*: prevalence, clinical significance, and transmission. Sex Transm Infect 2005;81:458–62.
16. Bjornelius E, Lidbrink P, Jensen JS. *Mycoplasma genitalium* in non-gonococcal urethritis–a study in Swedish male STD patients. Int J STD AIDS 2000;11:292–6.
17. Bradshaw CS, Tabrizi SN, Read TR, et al. Etiologies of nongonococcal urethritis: bacteria, viruses, and the association with orogenital exposure. J Infect Dis 2006;193:336–45.
18. Busolo F, Camposampiero D, Bordignon G, et al. Detection of *Mycoplasma genitalium* and *Chlamydia trachomatis* DNAs in male patients with urethritis using the polymerase chain reaction. New Microbiol 1997;20:325–32.
19. Deguchi T, Komeda H, Yasuda M, et al. *Mycoplasma genitalium* in non-gonococcal urethritis. Int J STD AIDS 1995;6:144–5.
20. Dupin N, Bijaoui G, Schwarzinger M, et al. Detection and quantification of *Mycoplasma genitalium* in male patients with urethritis. Clin Infect Dis 2003;37:602–5.
21. Falk L, Fredlund H, Jensen JS. Symptomatic urethritis is more prevalent in men infected with *Mycoplasma genitalium* than with *Chlamydia trachomatis*. Sex Transm Infect 2004;80:289–93.
22. Gambini D, Decleva I, Lupica L, et al. *Mycoplasma genitalium* in males with nongonococcal urethritis: prevalence and clinical efficacy of eradication. Sex Transm Dis 2000;27:226–9.
23. Horner P, Thomas B, Gilroy CB, et al. Role of *Mycoplasma genitalium* and *Ureaplasma urealyticum* in acute and chronic nongonococcal urethritis. Clin Infect Dis 2001;32:995–1003.
24. Horner PJ, Gilroy CB, Thomas BJ, et al. Association of *Mycoplasma genitalium* with acute non-gonococcal urethritis. Lancet 1993;342:582–5.
25. Iser P, Read TH, Tabrizi S, et al. Symptoms of non-gonococcal urethritis in heterosexual men: a case control study. Sex Transm Infect 2005;81:163–5.
26. Janier M, Lassau F, Casin I, et al. Male urethritis with and without discharge: a clinical and microbiological study. Sex Transm Dis 1995;22:244–52.
27. Jensen JS, Orsum R, Dohn B, et al. *Mycoplasma genitalium*: a cause of male urethritis? Genitourin Med 1993;69:265–9.
28. Johannisson G, Enstrom Y, Lowhagen GB, et al. Occurrence and treatment of *Mycoplasma genitalium* in patients visiting STD clinics in Sweden. Int J STD AIDS 2000;11:324–6.
29. Keane FE, Thomas BJ, Gilroy CB, et al. The association of *Mycoplasma hominis*, *Ureaplasma urealyticum* and *Mycoplasma genitalium* with bacterial vaginosis: observations on heterosexual women and their male partners. Int J STD AIDS 2000;11:356–60.
30. Leung A, Eastick K, Haddon LE, et al. *Mycoplasma genitalium* is associated with symptomatic urethritis. Int J STD AIDS 2006;17:285–8.

31. Maeda S, Deguchi T, Ishiko H, et al. Detection of *Mycoplasma genitalium*, *Mycoplasma hominis*, *Ureaplasma parvum* (biovar 1) and *Ureaplasma urealyticum* (biovar 2) in patients with non-gonococcal urethritis using polymerase chain reaction-microtiter plate hybridization. Int J Urol 2004;11:750–4.
32. Maeda S, Tamaki M, Nakano M, et al. Detection of *Mycoplasma genitalium* in patients with urethritis. J Urol 1998;159:405–7.
33. Mena L, Wang X, Mroczkowski TF, et al. *Mycoplasma genitalium* infections in asymptomatic men and men with urethritis attending a sexually transmitted diseases clinic in New Orleans. Clin Infect Dis 2002;35:1167–73.
34. Stamm WE, Batteiger BE, McCormack WM, et al. A randomized, double-blind study comparing single-dose rifalazil with single-dose azithromycin for the empirical treatment of nongonococcal urethritis in men. Sex Transm Dis 2007; 34:545–52.
35. Totten PA, Schwartz MA, Sjostrom KE, et al. Association of *Mycoplasma genitalium* with nongonococcal urethritis in heterosexual men. J Infect Dis 2001;183: 269–76.
36. Yoshida T, Deguchi T, Ito M, et al. Quantitative detection of *Mycoplasma genitalium* from first-pass urine of men with urethritis and asymptomatic men by real-time PCR. J Clin Microbiol 2002;40:1451–5.
37. Yu JT, Tang WY, Lau KH, et al. Asymptomatic urethral infection in male sexually transmitted disease clinic attendees. Int J STD AIDS 2008;19:155–8.
38. Berntsson M, Lowhagen GB, Bergstrom T, et al. Viral and bacterial aetiologies of male urethritis: findings of a high prevalence of Epstein-Barr virus. Int J STD AIDS 2010;21:191–4.
39. Couldwell DL, Gidding HF, Freedman EV, et al. *Ureaplasma urealyticum* is significantly associated with non-gonococcal urethritis in heterosexual Sydney men. Int J STD AIDS 2010;21:337–41.
40. Gaydos C, Maldeis NE, Hardick A, et al. *Mycoplasma genitalium* compared to chlamydia, gonorrhoea and trichomonas as an aetiological agent of urethritis in men attending STD clinics. Sex Transm Infect 2009;85:438–40.
41. Hilton J, Azariah S, Reid M. A case-control study of men with non-gonococcal urethritis at Auckland Sexual Health Service: rates of detection of *Mycoplasma genitalium*. Sex Health 2010;7:77–81.
42. Moi H, Reinton N, Moghaddam A. *Mycoplasma genitalium* is associated with symptomatic and asymptomatic non-gonococcal urethritis in men. Sex Transm Infect 2009;85:15–8.
43. Soni S, Alexander S, Verlander N, et al. The prevalence of urethral and rectal *Mycoplasma genitalium* and its associations in men who have sex with men attending a genitourinary medicine clinic. Sex Transm Infect 2010;86:21–4.
44. Taylor-Robinson D, Renton A, Jensen JS, et al. Association of *Mycoplasma genitalium* with acute non-gonococcal urethritis in Russian men: a comparison with gonococcal and chlamydial urethritis. Int J STD AIDS 2009;20:234–7.
45. Thurman AR, Musatovova O, Perdue S, et al. *Mycoplasma genitalium* symptoms, concordance and treatment in high-risk sexual dyads. Int J STD AIDS 2010;21:177–83.
46. Syvertsen L, Moghaddam A, Reinton N, et al. Etiology of non-gonococcal urethritis in men and its association with degree of urethritis. In: 27th Europe Congress of the International Union on Sexually Transmitted Infections. Antalya, Turkey, September 6–8, 2012. Abstract OP-20.
47. Uno M, Deguchi T, Komeda H, et al. Prevalence of *Mycoplasma genitalium* in men with gonococcal urethritis. Int J STD AIDS 1996;7:443–4.

48. Wetmore CM, Manhart LE, Lowens MS, et al. Characteristics associated with nongononcoccal urethritis among men with and without pathogens detected. In: CDC National STD Prevention Conference. Chicago, IL, USA, March 10–12, 2008. Abstract #A8d.
49. Sena AC, Lensing S, Rompalo A, et al. *Chlamydia trachomatis, Mycoplasma genitalium*, and *Trichomonas vaginalis* infections in men with nongonococcal urethritis: predictors and persistence after therapy. J Infect Dis 2012;206:357–65.
50. Hooton TM, Roberts MC, Roberts PL, et al. Prevalence of *Mycoplasma genitalium* determined by DNA probe in men with urethritis. Lancet 1988;1:266–8.
51. Wikstrom A, Jensen JS. *Mycoplasma genitalium*: a common cause of persistent urethritis among men treated with doxycycline. Sex Transm Infect 2006;82:276–9.
52. Yew HS, Anderson T, Coughlan E, et al. Induced macrolide resistance in *Mycoplasma genitalium* isolates from patients with recurrent nongonococcal urethritis. J Clin Microbiol 2011;49:1695–6.
53. Taylor-Robinson D, Gilroy CB, Thomas BJ, et al. *Mycoplasma genitalium* in chronic non-gonococcal urethritis. Int J STD AIDS 2004;15:21–5.
54. Eickhoff JH, Frimodt-Moller N, Walter S, et al. A double-blind, randomized, controlled multicentre study to compare the efficacy of ciprofloxacin with pivampicillin as oral therapy for epididymitis in men over 40 years of age. BJU Int 1999;84:827–34.
55. Ito S, Tsuchiya T, Yasuda M, et al. Prevalence of genital mycoplasmas and ureaplasmas in men younger than 40 years-of-age with acute epididymitis. Int J Urol 2012;19:234–8.
56. Hamasuna R. Acute epididymitis detected with *Mycoplasma genitalium*: a case report. Japanese J Sexually Transmitted Diseases 2008;19:89–92.
57. Bradshaw CS, Fairley CK, Lister NA, et al. *Mycoplasma genitalium* in men who have sex with men at male-only saunas. Sex Transm Infect 2009;85:432–5.
58. Edlund M, Blaxhult A, Bratt G. The spread of *Mycoplasma genitalium* among men who have sex with men. Int J STD AIDS 2012;23:455–6.
59. Francis SC, Kent CK, Klausner JD, et al. Prevalence of rectal *Trichomonas vaginalis* and *Mycoplasma genitalium* in male patients at the San Francisco STD clinic, 2005-2006. Sex Transm Dis 2008;35:797–800.
60. Taylor-Robinson D, Gilroy CB, Keane FE. Detection of several *Mycoplasma* species at various anatomical sites of homosexual men. Eur J Clin Microbiol Infect Dis 2003;22:291–3.
61. Brunham RC, Paavonen J, Stevens CE, et al. Mucopurulent cervicitis–the ignored counterpart in women of urethritis in men. N Engl J Med 1984;311:1–6.
62. Bjartling C, Osser S, Persson K. *Mycoplasma genitalium* in cervicitis and pelvic inflammatory disease among women at a gynecologic outpatient service. Am J Obstet Gynecol 2012;206(476):e1–8.
63. Casin I, Vexiau-Robert D, De La Salmoniere P, et al. High prevalence of *Mycoplasma genitalium* in the lower genitourinary tract of women attending a sexually transmitted disease clinic in Paris, France. Sex Transm Dis 2002;29:353–9.
64. Falk L. The overall agreement of proposed definitions of mucopurulent cervicitis in women at high risk of *Chlamydia* infection. Acta Derm Venereol 2010;90:506–11.
65. Falk L, Fredlund H, Jensen JS. Signs and symptoms of urethritis and cervicitis among women with or without *Mycoplasma genitalium* or *Chlamydia trachomatis* infection. Sex Transm Infect 2005;81:73–8.

66. Gaydos C, Maldeis NE, Hardick A, et al. *Mycoplasma genitalium* as a contributor to the multiple etiologies of cervicitis in women attending sexually transmitted disease clinics. Sex Transm Dis 2009;36(10):598–606.

67. Hogdahl M, Kihlstrom E. Leucocyte esterase testing of first-voided urine and urethral and cervical smears to identify *Mycoplasma genitalium*-infected men and women. Int J STD AIDS 2007;18:835–8.

68. Huppert JS, Mortensen JE, Reed JL, et al. *Mycoplasma genitalium* detected by transcription-mediated amplification is associated with *Chlamydia trachomatis* in adolescent women. Sex Transm Dis 2008;35:250–4.

69. Korte JE, Baseman JB, Cagle MP, et al. Cervicitis and genitourinary symptoms in women culture positive for *Mycoplasma genitalium*. Am J Reprod Immunol 2006;55:265–75.

70. Lusk MJ, Konecny P, Naing ZW, et al. *Mycoplasma genitalium* is associated with cervicitis and HIV infection in an urban Australian STI clinic population. Sex Transm Infect 2011;87:107–9.

71. Manhart LE, Critchlow CW, Holmes KK, et al. Mucopurulent cervicitis and *Mycoplasma genitalium*. J Infect Dis 2003;187:650–7.

72. Mobley VL, Hobbs MM, Lau K, et al. *Mycoplasma genitalium* infection in women attending a sexually transmitted infection clinic: diagnostic specimen type, coinfections, and predictors. Sex Transm Dis 2012;39:706–9.

73. Moi H, Reinton N, Moghaddam A. *Mycoplasma genitalium* in women with lower genital tract inflammation. Sex Transm Infect 2009;85:10–4.

74. Palmer HM, Gilroy CB, Claydon EJ, et al. Detection of *Mycoplasma genitalium* in the genitourinary tract of women by the polymerase chain reaction. Int J STD AIDS 1991;2:261–3.

75. Uno M, Deguchi T, Komeda H, et al. *Mycoplasma genitalium* in the cervices of Japanese women. Sex Transm Dis 1997;24:284–6.

76. Schlicht MJ, Lovrich SD, Sartin JS, et al. High prevalence of genital mycoplasmas among sexually active young adults with urethritis or cervicitis symptoms in La Crosse, Wisconsin. J Clin Microbiol 2004;42:4636–40.

77. Tosh AK, Van Der Pol B, Fortenberry JD, et al. *Mycoplasma genitalium* among adolescent women and their partners. J Adolesc Health 2007;40:412–7.

78. Vandepitte J, Bukenya J, Hughes P, et al. Clinical characteristics associated with *Mycoplasma genitalium* infection among women at high risk of HIV and other STI in Uganda. Sex Transm Dis 2012;39:487–91.

79. Eschenbach DA, Buchanan TM, Pollock HM, et al. Polymicrobial etiology of acute pelvic inflammatory disease. N Engl J Med 1975;293:166–71.

80. Soper DE. Pelvic inflammatory disease. Obstet Gynecol 2010;116:419–28.

81. Moller BR, Taylor-Robinson D, Furr PM. Serological evidence implicating *Mycoplasma genitalium* in pelvic inflammatory disease. Lancet 1984;1: 1102–3.

82. Lind K, Kristensen GB. Significance of antibodies to *Mycoplasma genitalium* in salpingitis. Eur J Clin Microbiol 1987;6:205–7.

83. Jurstrand M, Jensen JS, Magnuson A, et al. A serological study of the role of *Mycoplasma genitalium* in pelvic inflammatory disease and ectopic pregnancy. Sex Transm Infect 2007;83:319–23.

84. Cohen CR, Manhart LE, Bukusi EA, et al. Association between *Mycoplasma genitalium* and acute endometritis. Lancet 2002;359:765–6.

85. Haggerty CL, Totten PA, Astete SG, et al. Failure of cefoxitin and doxycycline to eradicate endometrial *Mycoplasma genitalium* and the consequence for clinical cure of pelvic inflammatory disease. Sex Transm Infect 2008;84:338–42.

86. Haggerty CL, Totten PA, Astete SG, et al. *Mycoplasma genitalium* among women with nongonococcal, nonchlamydial pelvic inflammatory disease. Infect Dis Obstet Gynecol 2006;2006:30184.

87. Wiesenfeld HC, Martin DH, Mancuso M, et al. The association between *Mycoplasma genitalium* and subclinical pelvic inflammatory disease. In: International Society for Sexually Transmitted Disease Research (ISSTDR). London, United Kingdom, June 28 - July 1, 2009. Abstract #P3.36.

88. Wiesenfeld HC. PID Abstract for ISSTDR - no title. In: 20th Meeting of the International Society for Sexually Transmitted Diseases Research (ISSTDR). Vienna, Austria, July 14–17, 2013.

89. Simms I, Eastick K, Mallinson H, et al. Associations between *Mycoplasma genitalium, Chlamydia trachomatis*, and pelvic inflammatory disease. Sex Transm Infect 2003;79:154–6.

90. Cohen CR, Mugo NR, Astete SG, et al. Detection of *Mycoplasma genitalium* in women with laparoscopically diagnosed acute salpingitis. Sex Transm Infect 2005;81:463–6.

91. Bjartling C, Osser S, Persson K. The association between *Mycoplasma genitalium* and pelvic inflammatory disease after termination of pregnancy. BJOG 2010;117:361–4.

92. Oakeshott P, Aghaizu A, Hay P, et al. Is *Mycoplasma genitalium* in women the "New Chlamydia?" A community-based prospective cohort study. Clin Infect Dis 2010;51:1160–6.

93. Taylor-Robinson D, Jensen JS, Svenstrup H, et al. Difficulties experienced in defining the microbial cause of pelvic inflammatory disease. Int J STD AIDS 2012;23:18–24.

94. Moller BR, Taylor-Robinson D, Furr PM, et al. Acute upper genital-tract disease in female monkeys provoked experimentally by *Mycoplasma genitalium.* Br J Exp Pathol 1985;66:417–26.

95. Short VL, Totten PA, Ness RB, et al. Clinical presentation of *Mycoplasma genitalium* infection versus *Neisseria gonorrhoeae* infection among women with pelvic inflammatory disease. Clin Infect Dis 2009;48:41–7.

96. Clausen HF, Fedder J, Drasbek M, et al. Serological investigation of *Mycoplasma genitalium* in infertile women. Hum Reprod 2001;16:1866–74.

97. Svenstrup HF, Fedder J, Kristoffersen SE, et al. *Mycoplasma genitalium, Chlamydia trachomatis*, and tubal factor infertility–a prospective study. Fertil Steril 2008;90:513–20.

98. Grzesko J, Elias M, Maczynska B, et al. Occurrence of *Mycoplasma genitalium* in fertile and infertile women. Fertil Steril 2009;91(6):2376–80.

99. Gdoura R, Kchaou W, Ammar-Keskes L, et al. Assessment of *Chlamydia trachomatis, Ureaplasma urealyticum, Ureaplasma parvum, Mycoplasma hominis,* and *Mycoplasma genitalium* in semen and first void urine specimens of asymptomatic male partners of infertile couples. J Androl 2008;29:198–206.

100. Gdoura R, Kchaou W, Chaari C, et al. *Ureaplasma urealyticum, Ureaplasma parvum, Mycoplasma hominis* and *Mycoplasma genitalium* infections and semen quality of infertile men. BMC Infect Dis 2007;7:129.

101. Lu GC, Schwebke JR, Duffy LB, et al. Midtrimester vaginal *Mycoplasma genitalium* in women with subsequent spontaneous preterm birth. Am J Obstet Gynecol 2001;185:163–5.

102. Labbe AC, Frost E, Deslandes S, et al. *Mycoplasma genitalium* is not associated with adverse outcomes of pregnancy in Guinea-Bissau. Sex Transm Infect 2002; 78:289–91.

103. Oakeshott P, Hay P, Taylor-Robinson D, et al. Prevalence of *Mycoplasma genitalium* in early pregnancy and relationship between its presence and pregnancy outcome. BJOG 2004;111:1464–7.

104. Kataoka S, Yamada T, Chou K, et al. Association between preterm birth and vaginal colonization by mycoplasmas in early pregnancy. J Clin Microbiol 2006;44:51–5.

105. Edwards RK, Ferguson RJ, Reyes L, et al. Assessing the relationship between preterm delivery and various microorganisms recovered from the lower genital tract. J Matern Fetal Neonatal Med 2006;19:357–63.

106. Hitti J, Garcia P, Totten P, et al. Correlates of cervical *Mycoplasma genitalium* and risk of preterm birth among Peruvian women. Sex Transm Dis 2010;37:81–5.

107. Short VL, Jensen JS, Nelson DB, et al. *Mycoplasma genitalium* among young, urban pregnant women. Infect Dis Obstet Gynecol 2010;2010:984760.

108. Napierala Mavedzenge S, Weiss HA. Association of *Mycoplasma genitalium* and HIV infection: a systematic review and meta-analysis. AIDS 2009;23:611–20.

109. Manhart LE, Mostad SB, Baeten JM, et al. High *Mycoplasma genitalium* organism burden is associated with shedding of HIV-1 DNA from the cervix. J Infect Dis 2008;197:733–6.

110. Manhas A, Sethi S, Sharma M, et al. Association of genital mycoplasmas including *Mycoplasma genitalium* in HIV infected men with nongonococcal urethritis attending STD & HIV clinics. Indian J Med Res 2009;129:305–10.

111. Mansson F, Camara C, Biai A, et al. High prevalence of HIV-1, HIV-2 and other sexually transmitted infections among women attending two sexual health clinics in Bissau, Guinea-Bissau, West Africa. Int J STD AIDS 2010;21:631–5.

112. Mhlongo S, Magooa P, Muller EE, et al. Etiology and STI/HIV coinfections among patients with urethral and vaginal discharge syndromes in South Africa. Sex Transm Dis 2010;37:566–70.

113. Gatski M, Martin DH, Theall K, et al. *Mycoplasma genitalium* infection among HIV-positive women: prevalence, risk factors and association with vaginal shedding. Int J STD AIDS 2011;22:155–9.

114. Mavedzenge SN, Muller EE, Lewis DA, et al. Epidemiology of *Mycoplasma genitalium* and genital HIV-1 RNA – a longitudinal study among HIV-infected Zimbabwean women. In: 19th Meeting of the International Society for STD Research (ISSTDR). Quebec City, Quebec, Canada, July 10–13, 2011. Abstract P1-S.57.

115. Johnston LG, Paz-Bailey G, Morales-Miranda S, et al. High prevalence of *Mycoplasma genitalium* among female sex workers in Honduras: implications for the spread of HIV and other sexually transmitted infections. Int J STD AIDS 2012;23:5–11.

116. Mavedzenge SN, Van Der Pol B, Weiss HA, et al. The association between *Mycoplasma genitalium* and HIV-1 acquisition in African women. AIDS 2012;26:617–24.

117. Vandepitte J, Weiss HA, Bukenya J, et al. Alcohol use, *Mycoplasma genitalium*, and other STIs associated with HIV incidence among women at high risk in Kampala, Uganda. J Acquir Immune Defic Syndr 2013;62:119–26.

118. Bjornelius E, Anagrius C, Bojs G, et al. *Mycoplasma genitalium*: when to test and treat. Present status in Scandinavia. In: 15th Meeting of the International Society for STD Research (ISSTDR) Ottawa, Ontario, Canada. July 27–30, 2003. Abstract O388.

119. Falk L, Fredlund H, Jensen JS. Tetracycline treatment does not eradicate *Mycoplasma genitalium*. Sex Transm Infect 2003;79:318–9.

120. Schwebke JR, Rompalo A, Taylor S, et al. Re-evaluating the treatment of nongonococcal urethritis: emphasizing emerging pathogens–a randomized clinical trial. Clin Infect Dis 2011;52:163–70.
121. Manhart LE, Gillespie CW, Lowens MS, et al. Standard treatment regimens for nongonococcal urethritis have similar but declining cure rates: a randomized controlled trial. Clin Infect Dis 2013;56(7):934–42.
122. Bradshaw CS, Chen MY, Fairley CK. Persistence of *Mycoplasma genitalium* following azithromycin therapy. PLoS One 2008;3:e3618.
123. Bradshaw CS, Jensen JS, Tabrizi SN, et al. Azithromycin failure in *Mycoplasma genitalium* urethritis. Emerg Infect Dis 2006;12:1149–52.
124. Jernberg E, Moghaddam A, Moi H. Azithromycin and moxifloxacin for microbiological cure of *Mycoplasma genitalium* infection: an open study. Int J STD AIDS 2008;19:676–9.
125. Terada M, Izumi K, Ohki E, et al. Antimicrobial efficacies of several antibiotics against uterine cervicitis caused by *Mycoplasma genitalium*. J Infect Chemother 2012;18:313–7.
126. Twin J, Jensen JS, Bradshaw CS, et al. Transmission and selection of macrolide resistant *Mycoplasma genitalium* infections detected by rapid high resolution melt analysis. PLoS One 2012;7:e35593.
127. Walker J, Fairley CK, Bradshaw CS, et al. *Mycoplasma genitalium* incidence, organism load and treatment failure among a cohort of young Australian women. Clin Infect Dis 2013;56(8):1094–100.
128. Anagrius C, Lore B, Jensen JS. Treatment of *Mycoplasma genitalium*. Observations from a Swedish STD clinic. PLoS One 2013;8:e61481.
129. Gesink DC, Mulvad G, Montgomery-Andersen R, et al. *Mycoplasma genitalium* presence, resistance and epidemiology in Greenland. Int J Circumpolar Health 2012;71:1–8.
130. Ross JD, Cronje HS, Paszkowski T, et al. Moxifloxacin versus ofloxacin plus metronidazole in uncomplicated pelvic inflammatory disease: results of a multicentre, double blind, randomised trial. Sex Transm Infect 2006;82:446–51.

Pelvic Inflammatory Disease
Current Concepts in Pathogenesis, Diagnosis and Treatment

Caroline Mitchell, MD, MPH*, Malavika Prabhu, MD

KEYWORDS

- Pelvic inflammatory disease • *Neisseria gonorrhoeae* • *Chlamydia trachomatis*
- Cervical infection

KEY POINTS

- The diagnosis of pelvic inflammatory disease (PID) is based on clinical findings and requires a high index of suspicion.
- PID is caused both by common sexually transmitted infections, such as *Neisseria gonorrhoeae* and *Chlamydia trachomatis*, and by anaerobic vaginal microbes.
- Antibiotic coverage for anaerobic bacteria should be considered when treating severe PID.
- Early identification and treatment of cervical infections can prevent PID.

Pelvic inflammatory disease (PID) is characterized by infection and inflammation of the upper genital tract in women: the uterus, fallopian tubes, and/or ovaries. Although a definitive diagnosis of PID can be made by laparoscopic visualization of inflamed, purulent fallopian tubes, PID is generally a clinical diagnosis and thus represents a diagnostic challenge. Because PID can cause significant reproductive health sequelae for women, diagnosis and treatment algorithms advise a high index of suspicion for PID in any woman of reproductive age with pelvic or abdominal pain, and err on the side of recommending what likely amounts to overtreatment with antibiotic regimens.

EPIDEMIOLOGY

In the United States in 2000, there were an estimated 1.2 million medical visits for PID,[1] a number that has been decreasing since 1985.[2–4] This decrease is attributed in part to widespread adoption of screening for *Chlamydia trachomatis*, the goal of which is to identify and treat asymptomatic cases of cervicitis before they can progress to PID.[5]

Department of Obstetrics & Gynecology, University of Washington, 1959 NE Pacific Street, Seattle, WA 98195, USA
* Corresponding author. Harborview Women's Clinic, 325 9th Avenue, Box 359865, Seattle, WA 98105.
E-mail address: camitch@uw.edu

Infect Dis Clin N Am 27 (2013) 793–809
http://dx.doi.org/10.1016/j.idc.2013.08.004
0891-5520/13/$ – see front matter © 2013 Elsevier Inc. All rights reserved.

id.theclinics.com

Estimated direct medical costs associated with PID and its sequelae (ectopic pregnancy, chronic pelvic pain, and tubal infertility) were as high as US$1.88 billion in 1998, even though most women receive care as outpatients.[6]

Risk factors for PID are the same as those for acquisition of sexually transmitted diseases: multiple sexual partners, young age, smoking, and illicit drug use.[6–9] Douching has been implicated in some studies, and has been observed to double a woman's risk of upper genital tract infection.[8,10,11] Oral contraceptive use has been associated with lower rates of clinical PID, although it is not clear whether this is due to fewer infections or fewer symptoms, and thus underdiagnosis.[12–14] Bacterial vaginosis (BV) has also been associated with PID, though primarily in cross-sectional studies unable to determine causality.[15] In the prospective Gyn Infections Follow-Through study (GIFT), women with BV at enrollment did not have higher risk for PID over 4 years of follow-up, although women with *Neisseria gonorrhoeae* and *C trachomatis* did.[16]

ETIOLOGY

In early studies of PID, *N gonorrhoeae* was the most commonly isolated pathogen, and is still more likely than other pathogens to cause severe symptoms.[13,17–19] However, as the prevalence of gonorrhea has decreased, its importance as a causal agent for PID has diminished.[20,21] *C trachomatis* remains a significant pathogen associated with PID, detected in up to 60% of women with confirmed salpingitis or endometritis.[22–24] *Mycoplasma genitalium* has been independently associated with PID, although its prevalence is low in most populations that have been studied (this is further discussed in the article by Manhart elsewhere in this issue).[25,26] The proportion of cases of PID that involve nongonococcal, nonchlamydial etiology ranges between 9% and 23% in women with confirmed salpingitis or endometritis, even as diagnostic testing for gonorrhea and chlamydia become more sensitive.[7,22,24,27,28] In these cases, the microbial community is often diverse and includes anaerobes such as *Peptostreptococcus* spp and *Prevotella* spp.[23,27] Even in women with gonorrhea or chlamydia, detection of anaerobes in the upper genital tract is frequent and is associated with more severe disease.[16,22] In a study of Kenyan women with laparoscopically confirmed salpingitis, polymerase chain reaction assay of tubal samples for the bacterial 16S rRNA gene identified multiple species, including several associated with BV such as *Atopobium vaginae*, *Leptotrichia* spp, *Peptostreptococcus* spp, and *Prevotella* spp.[29]

PATHOGENESIS

Mathematical modeling based on epidemiologic and microbiologic studies suggests that 8% to 10% of women with *C trachomatis* infection will develop PID if not treated,[30] although in studies that followed women with chlamydial endocervical infection without treatment, the rate was even lower.[31,32] When both the lower and upper genital tract are sampled there is a clear gradient of infections, with a higher proportion of women testing positive at the vagina and/or cervix, fewer in the endometrium, and less frequently in the fallopian tubes.[23,24,27] One component of protection from bacterial ascent is the physical barrier of the cervix and its mucus barrier. Endometrial detection of gonorrhea or chlamydia is more frequent in the proliferative phase of the menstrual cycle[18] when cervical mucus is thinner[33] and the peristaltic contractions of the uterus move fluid cephalad.[34] There is also likely an immunologic component to the cervical barrier; genetic polymorphisms in toll-like receptor (TLR) genes seem to increase the risk of upper genital tract infection,[24] as do certain human leukocyte antigen class II alleles, suggesting that individual differences in immune function may increase the risk of developing PID in the setting of cervical infection.

Tubal damage is best described in the context of chlamydial infection, and appears to be related both to an innate immune inflammatory response initiated by the epithelial cells infected by C trachomatis[35] and to an adaptive T-cell response.[36,37] Although antibody titers to chlamydial antigens are increased in severe disease,[38,39] higher titers have not been associated with worse reproductive outcomes.[40] In human studies, evaluation of tubal inflammation is difficult without surgical intervention; thus, many studies use endometritis as a marker for tubal inflammation. Kiviat and colleagues[41] correlated the presence of both neutrophils and plasma cells in endometrial biopsies with visible salpingitis. In a cohort of women with mild to moderate PID who were treated with broad-spectrum antibiotics, the presence of either neutrophils or plasma cells in an endometrial biopsy was not associated with decreased fertility.[42] Plasma cells alone were found in 33% of endometrial samples of low-risk women[43] and were not associated with laparoscopic abnormalities; however, in women at high risk of sexually transmitted infections, plasma cell endometritis appears to be associated with decreased fertility.[44] The heterogeneity of these findings suggests that there is a range of individual immune response to upper genital tract infection, and that not all women have the same likelihood of reproductive sequelae from PID.

CLINICAL EVALUATION AND DIFFERENTIAL DIAGNOSIS

In practical terms, when a sexually active woman presents to the clinic or emergency department with lower abdominal or pelvic pain, PID must be considered in the differential diagnosis, which also includes appendicitis, ectopic pregnancy, ovarian torsion, intrapelvic bleeding, rupture of an adnexal mass, endometriosis, and gastroenteritis.[45] Key components of the physical examination include:

1. Abdominal examination, including palpation of the right upper quadrant
2. Vaginal speculum examination, including inspection of the cervix for friability and mucopurulent cervical discharge
3. Bimanual examination, assessing for cervical motion, uterine or adnexal tenderness, and pelvic masses
4. Microscopic evaluation of a sample of cervicovaginal discharge to assess for Trichomonas vaginalis, BV, and/or leukorrhea

The clinical presentation of PID is variable (**Table 1**), so a high index of suspicion is necessary. Symptoms may differ depending on the pathogens responsible. In the PID Evaluation and Clinical Health (PEACH) trial, women with PID associated with C trachomatis or M genitalium took almost 1 week longer to present to care than women with gonorrhea-associated PID, suggesting milder symptoms.[19] Women with gonococcal

Table 1		
Prevalence of signs and symptoms in women with confirmed salpingitis or endometritis		
Symptom	**Prevalence (%)**	**Reference**
Temperature >38.5°C	33–34	47,49
WBC >10,000 cells/mL	36–70	49,50
ESR >15 mm/h	36–77	49,50
Mucopurulent cervical discharge	56	49
Leukorrhea (≥10 WBC/hpf on wet mount)	22.1	53
Irregular vaginal bleeding	36–64	47,50

Abbreviations: ESR, erythrocyte sedimentation rate; hpf, high-power field; WBC, white blood cells.

infection are more likely to have fever, adnexal tenderness, mucopurulent cervicitis, and an elevated peripheral white blood cell (WBC) count.[46]

SENSITIVITY AND SPECIFICITY OF CDC DIAGNOSTIC CRITERIA

The clinical diagnosis of PID is based on recommendations from the Centers for Disease Control and Prevention (CDC). Minimum diagnostic criteria (**Box 1**) have been set with a high sensitivity and low specificity in order to detect as many cases of clinical disease as possible, thus potentially avoiding the long-term reproductive sequelae and economic costs associated with delayed diagnosis and lack of treatment.

In a cohort of patients with suspected PID who underwent laparoscopy in Lund, Sweden, PID was considered when a patient presented with lower abdominal pain and at least 2 of the following: abnormal vaginal discharge, fever, vomiting, menstrual irregularities, urinary symptoms, proctitis symptoms, marked tenderness of the pelvic organs on bimanual examination, palpable adnexal mass, or erythrocyte sedimentation rate (ESR) greater than 15 mm/h. Only 65% of women suspected to have PID using these criteria actually had salpingitis.[47] A 2003 reanalysis of data from this cohort demonstrated that the combination of fever (temperature >38.3°C), elevated ESR, and adnexal tenderness achieved the highest combination of sensitivity and specificity, 65% and 66%, respectively, for acute salpingitis.[48] In other words, these criteria would have a 35% false-negative rate for predicting laparoscopically determined PID.

It is difficult to calculate the exact sensitivity and specificity of the CDC diagnostic criteria, as there at least 2 potential gold standards for a true positive diagnosis of PID: salpingitis at laparoscopy or endometritis on endometrial biopsy. Because laparoscopy is expensive, invasive, and not part of a standard evaluation of PID, many

---

Box 1
CDC criteria for PID diagnosis

Minimum Criteria (At Least 1 Needed for Diagnosis)	Additional Criteria (Support a Diagnosis of PID)	Definitive Criteria (Confirm the Diagnosis of PID)
• Cervical motion tenderness • Uterine tenderness • Adnexal tenderness	• Oral temperature higher than 101°F/38.3°C • Abnormal vaginal or cervical discharge • White blood cells on saline wet mount (>10 polymorphonuclear leukocytes per high-power field[101]) • Elevated erythrocyte sedimentation rate (>15 mm/h) • Elevated C-reactive protein • Elevated white blood cell count higher than 10,000 cells/mL • Laboratory evidence of *Neisseria gonorrhoeae* or *Chlamydia trachomatis* infection	• Histopathologic evidence of endometritis • Imaging showing thickened, fluid-filled tubes, with or without pelvic free fluid or tubo-ovarian complex • Doppler studies suggesting pelvic infection • Intra-abdominal findings consistent with PID on laparoscopy

Adapted from Workowski KA, Berman S. Sexually transmitted diseases treatment guidelines, 2010. MMWR Recomm Rep 2010;59(RR-12):1–110.

studies use endometritis as a marker of upper genital tract infection and inflammation. Endometritis and salpingitis are correlated; histologic endometritis has sensitivity of 89% to 92% and specificity of 63% to 87% for laparoscopically diagnosed acute salpingitis, with only 7% to 22% of patients with clinically suspected PID having salpingitis without endometritis.[28,41,49,50] However, whereas the presence and severity of salpingitis is correlated with a risk of ectopic pregnancy and infertility,[21] endometritis is not as consistently associated with these outcomes[42]; this may be because not all women with endometritis have salpingitis (**Table 2**), thus diluting the association.

LABORATORY TESTING

Because PID is a clinical diagnosis, laboratory data or imaging studies are not usually necessary, but can be helpful in establishing the diagnosis or in defining its severity.[51] In the PEACH trial, which enrolled women with abdominal pain, pelvic tenderness, and evidence of lower genital tract inflammation, an elevated leukocyte count ($\geq$10,000 cells/mL) had 41% sensitivity and 76% specificity for the presence of endometritis.[52] The presence of 1 or more neutrophils per 1000× field saline wet mount of vaginal discharge had 91% sensitivity and 26.3% specificity for endometritis.[53] In another cohort study, an elevated ESR (>15 mm/h) had 70% sensitivity and 52% specificity for endometritis or salpingitis. Elevated WBC had 57% sensitivity and 88% specificity, whereas the presence of increased numbers of vaginal neutrophils ($\geq$3 per high-power field) had 78% sensitivity and 39% specificity.[54] In a cohort of women at high risk for pelvic infections, absence of vaginal WBCs had excellent negative predictive value (95%).[53] These data suggest that if an evaluation of a saline microscopy of vaginal fluid reveals no WBCs (leukorrhea), an alternative diagnosis to PID should be considered.

IMAGING STUDIES

Ultrasonography can also be used to aid in the diagnosis of PID and its direct treatment. A finding of thickened, fluid-filled tubes has 85% sensitivity and 100% specificity for endometritis among women with clinically diagnosed PID.[55] Timor-Tritsch and colleagues[56] detailed the various transvaginal sonographic markers of acute tubal inflammatory disease, including dilated tubal shape, abnormal wall structure, increased wall thickness ($\geq$5 mm), and presence of pelvic peritoneal fluid (free fluid or inclusion cyst). In a study comparing 30 patients with clinical PID confirmed with laparoscopy and 20 normal women, power Doppler demonstrating tubal hyperemia was 100% sensitive and 80% specific for PID; in addition, altered tubal shape, structure, and wall thickness were seen in an overwhelming majority of patients with pyosalpinx.[57] Magnetic resonance imaging, with its highly sensitive and specific ability to identify thickened,

Table 2
Incidence of endometritis and salpingitis among women with suspected PID and both laparoscopic and endometrial evaluation

Authors,[Ref.] Year	Endometritis Alone	Salpingitis Alone	Endometritis + Salpingitis
Paavonen et al,[102] 1985	3/27 (11.1%)	2/27 (7.4%)	16/27 (59.3%)
Wasserheit et al,[28] 1986	8/33 (24.2%)	1/33 (3.0%)	14/33 (42.4%)
Eckert et al,[49] 2002	26/152 (17.1%)	11/144 (7.6%)	64/144 (44.4%)

fluid-filled tubes, pyosalpinx, pelvic free fluid, and tubo-ovarian abscess (TOA), has also been proposed as a diagnostic modality for PID; however, it is very costly and not easily accessible or applicable to women seeking outpatient evaluation for possible PID.[58]

INPATIENT VERSUS OUTPATIENT MANAGEMENT

The therapeutic goal for the treatment of PID is 2-fold: short-term microbiologic and clinical cure; and long-term prevention of sequelae, namely tubal infertility, ectopic pregnancy, and chronic pelvic pain. Since the 1980s, PID therapy has shifted from the inpatient to the outpatient setting, with a 68% decline in hospitalization[4] attributable in part to several studies showing equivalent short-term outcomes with outpatient versus inpatient therapy for mild to moderate PID.[59,60] Between 1995 and 2001, 89% of all PID visits occurred in the ambulatory setting.[4] Current criteria for inpatient hospitalization are summarized in **Box 2**.

The PEACH trial compared inpatient administration of parenteral cefoxitin and doxycycline (parenteral/oral) with outpatient administration of intramuscular cefoxitin and oral doxycycline, and found no short-term (30-day) differences in microbiologic or clinical cure[61] or long-term differences in reproductive health outcomes (**Table 3**).[62] A secondary analysis among participants of the PEACH trial also found no long-term outcome differences by treatment group among those with clinically confirmed endometritis or upper genital tract gonorrheal or chlamydial infection.[61,62] Of interest, a representative subpopulation from PEACH revealed a 70% mean treatment adherence rate, with only 17% of participants taking doxycycline exactly as prescribed.[63] Similar rates of poor adherence to doxycycline or tetracycline prescribed for outpatient therapy for sexually transmitted infections (STIs) have been seen, particularly in the setting of gastrointestinal side effects.[64,65] This finding may explain the relatively high rates of ongoing disease and long-term sequelae in the PEACH cohort.

Whereas many of the original efficacy studies mandated inpatient intravenous treatment of 48 to 96 hours before switching to oral therapy,[61,66] current practice is to treat with intravenous medications until there is clinical improvement for 24 hours or more. However, because intravenous doxycycline can cause significant phlebitis and its oral bioavailability is comparable with that of parenteral bioavailability, an earlier switch to oral doxycycline can be made if a patient is tolerating oral medications.[61]

CDC RECOMMENDATIONS FOR ANTIMICROBIAL THERAPY

Current recommendations for antimicrobial treatment regimens in PID were published in 2010 (**Table 4**), and are scheduled for update in 2014.[67] A guiding principle for selection of antimicrobial therapy for PID is that the regimen should cover *N gonorrhoeae*

Box 2
Criteria for inpatient management of PID

- Surgical emergencies cannot be ruled out
- Pregnancy
- Lack of clinical response to oral antimicrobial PID therapy after 72 hours
- Inability to tolerate or comply with outpatient management
- Severe illness, high fever, nausea, vomiting
- Presence of tubo-ovarian abscess

Table 3
Summary of short-term and long-term effects of outpatient compared with inpatient therapy for mild to moderate PID in the PEACH trial

	Outpatient (%)	Inpatient (%)	P Value
Short Term (30 d)			
Gonorrhea positive	3.9	2.4	.44
Chlamydia positive	2.7	3.6	.52
Persistent tenderness	20.6	18.4	.50
Endometritis	45.9	37.6	.09
Long Term (mean 35 mo)			
Pregnancy	59.4	55.6	NS
Ectopic	1.2	0.2	NS
Infertility	16.7	20.6	NS
Chronic pelvic pain	40.7	44.6	NS
Recurrent PID	18.4	24.3	NS

Abbreviation: NS, not statistically significant.

Adapted from Ness RB, Soper DE, Holley RL, et al. Effectiveness of inpatient and outpatient treatment strategies for women with pelvic inflammatory disease: results from the Pelvic Inflammatory Disease Evaluation and Clinical Health (PEACH) randomized trial. Am J Obstet Gynecol 2002;186(5):929–37; and Ness RB, Trautmann G, Richter HE, et al. Effectiveness of treatment strategies of some women with pelvic inflammatory disease: a randomized trial. Obstet Gynecol 2005;106(3):573–80.

and *C trachomatis*, regardless of results of diagnostic testing for these pathogens. Therapy for gonorrhea, and therefore PID, shifted away from fluoroquinolone-based regimens between the 2006 and 2010 iterations of the CDC Treatment Guidelines, given the rapid emergence of fluoroquinolone resistance.[68] In 2012, after reports of increasing prevalence of cefixime-resistant gonorrhea, the guidelines were changed again to drop cefixime as one of the first-line outpatient treatment options for cervicitis.[69] With additional cephalosporin resistance to gonorrhea reported, as discussed in the article by Barbee and Dombrowski elsewhere in this issue, the potential for development of resistance that could compromise treatment of gonorrhea-associated PID is of great concern.

ALTERNATIVE ANTIMICROBIAL REGIMENS

Although not part of the CDC recommendations, newer data suggest that parenteral followed by oral azithromycin, either as monotherapy or in combination with doxycycline and metronidazole, produces clinical cure rates of 97% to 98% at 2 weeks after initiation of treatment, and microbiologic cure rates of 90% to 94% at 6 weeks posttreatment.[70] The azithromycin-based regimens were compared with third-generation cephalosporin-based regimens or parenteral amoxicillin-based regimens and showed no statistically significant difference in clinical or microbiologic cure rates, although the study had a high dropout rate and low proportion of anaerobic bacteria isolated from endocervix and endometrium.[70] Another trial compared intramuscular ceftriaxone plus oral azithromycin with the standard of oral doxycycline, and found higher rates of clinical and histologic cure with azithromycin, although rates of cure in both arms were less than 80%.[71]

M genitalium is neither tested for nor considered when choosing therapy. However, newer evidence suggests a greater than 4-fold higher risk of treatment failure with

Table 4
Reported efficacy of CDC-recommended treatment regimens for inpatient and outpatient management of PID

	Response to Treatment (%)	Reference
Inpatient		
Cefotetan 2 g IV q 12 h AND Doxycycline 100 mg PO/IV q 12 h[a,b] Followed by doxycycline 100 mg PO BID for a total of 14 d	89–94	66,103
Cefoxitin 2 g IV q 6 h AND Doxycycline 100 mg PO/IV q 12 h[a,b] Followed by doxycycline 100 mg PO BID for a total of 14 d	84–95	61,103–106
Clindamycin 900 mg IV q 8 h AND Gentamicin 2 mg/kg IV/IM load then 1.5 mg/kg maintenance OR 3–5 mg/kg daily dosing Followed by doxycycline 100 mg PO BID OR Clindamycin 450 mg PO QID,[c] total 14-d course	84–90	66,104,106
Ampicillin/sulbactam 3 g IV q 6 h AND Doxycycline 100 mg PO/IV q 12 h[a,b] Followed by doxycycline 100 mg PO BID, total 14-d course	85–94[d]	71,105
Outpatient[e]		
Ceftriaxone 250 mg IM once AND Doxycycline 100 mg PO BID, total 14 d	72–95	60,70,107
Cefoxitin 2 mg IM once, with probenecid 1 g PO once AND Doxycycline 100 mg PO BID, total 14 d	90	61
Other parenteral third-generation cephalosporin (cefotaxime, ceftizoxime) AND Doxycycline 100 mg PO BID, total 14 d	—	—

Abbreviations: BID, twice daily; IM, intramuscular; IV, intravenous; PO, by mouth; q, every; QID, 4 times daily.

[a] Equivalent oral and IV bioavailability for doxycycline. IV doxycycline causes burning, therefore elect for oral doxycycline if able to be tolerated.

[b] Must add clindamycin 450 mg PO QID or metronidazole 500 mg PO q 6 h in the setting of tubo-ovarian abscess, for a total 14-day course.

[c] Continue clindamycin in the setting of tubo-ovarian abscess.

[d] Higher end of range is a regimen including metronidazole.

[e] For all 3 regimens, consider adding metronidazole 500 mg PO BID for 7 days.

a cefoxitin/doxycycline regimen when *M genitalium* is present, although there were no differences in reproductive sequelae or recurrent PID, as discussed in the article by Manhart elsewhere in this issue.[72] Doxycycline has poor efficacy against *M genitalium* (cure rates from 17% to 94%), and although azithromycin is more effective (67%–100% cure), moxifloxacin seems to be the most effective treatment.[73] In cases of persistent PID not responsive to standard therapy, testing for and treatment of *M genitalium* should be considered, and presumptive therapy with moxifloxacin may be warranted.

ANAEROBES: TO COVER OR NOT?

There is little clarity on the need for empiric coverage for anaerobic bacteria when PID is diagnosed, in part because there is a lack of clear understanding of the contribution of anaerobes to pathogenesis in PID. Several studies have shown that BV is associated with PID, with BV-associated anaerobic bacteria present in endometritis, but that BV may not actually cause acute PID.[16,61,74] However, other data have not shown any long-term reproductive sequelae of histologically diagnosed anaerobic endometritis, even when treatment with a cephalosporin-based regimen with poor anaerobic coverage was provided.[42] Few studies have specifically examined microbiologic cure rates of antimicrobial treatment regimens targeting anaerobic bacteria. Some BV-associated microbes may form a biofilm on the endometrial surface, which could limit the ability of antibiotics to eliminate colonization.[75] The CDC currently recommends consideration of treatment regimens with anaerobic coverage until data suggest equivalent prevention of reproductive sequelae in treatment regimens lacking anaerobic coverage.[67] Anaerobic coverage should be included in women with a TOA and with BV, regardless of the latter's potential etiologic role in the development of acute PID.[67,76]

ADDITIONAL TREATMENT CONSIDERATIONS

Among patients who qualified for outpatient therapy, reevaluation of clinical status should occur within 72 hours, or sooner if indicated. If no meaningful clinical response is detected, patients with PID may require inpatient hospitalization, transition to parenteral antibiotics, further diagnostic tests including additional laboratory studies and imaging to evaluate for possible TOA, and possible surgical intervention.

Empiric treatment of gonorrhea and chlamydia is recommended for all male sexual partners within the past 60 days, or the most recent sexual partner if more than 60 days ago, regardless of symptoms or the result of gonorrhea and chlamydia testing in the female patient with PID.[67] Women diagnosed with PID should be offered a test for human immunodeficiency virus (HIV) at the time of diagnosis. Repeat testing for gonorrhea or chlamydia in 3 to 6 months is recommended if initial testing is positive for either infection.[67]

TUBO-OVARIAN ABSCESS

Although the presenting signs and symptoms of a TOA are not often distinct from those with salpingitis/endometritis, there are often more objective signs of infection and inflammation. A large series of patients with ultrasonographically or surgically confirmed TOA found that 60% had a temperature higher than 37.8°C, 68% had leukocytosis (>10,000 cells/mL), 26% had nausea, and 19% had chronic abdominopelvic pain.[77] In women with PID, palpation of an adnexal mass on physical examination, significant pain limiting proper evaluation of the adnexa, severe illness, or lack of clinical response to antimicrobial therapy should prompt imaging studies. In addition, imaging can help to evaluate for alternative diagnoses such as appendicitis, ovarian torsion, or cyst rupture.

Inpatient observation is recommended for at least 24 hours among hemodynamically stable women with a TOA, with the aim of observing for early signs of sepsis or potential abscess rupture. Surgical exploration on initial evaluation is indicated in the setting of an acute abdomen and signs of sepsis or hemodynamic instability, particularly if a ruptured TOA is suspected. Antimicrobial therapy should be parenteral to begin with, and should include clindamycin or metronidazole to cover anaerobes.[67] Antimicrobial therapy alone, with appropriate anaerobic coverage and the ability to penetrate and function in abscess cavities, is effective in 70% to 84% of women.[77,78]

In one cohort of women admitted with TOA, 60% of those with an abscess larger than 10 cm needed surgical management, compared with 20% of those with abscesses of 4 to 6 cm.[78] When no clinical improvement is noted within 72 hours of antibiotic initiation, minimally invasive drainage of the abscess or surgical management can be pursued; however, significant clinical deterioration at any time usually indicates the need for surgical exploration.[77] A study of empiric transvaginal ultrasound-guided aspiration of

TOAs at the time of diagnosis, in concert with antimicrobial therapy, revealed that the procedure is safe and well tolerated, and averted surgical management in 93% of cases.[79,80]

SPECIAL POPULATIONS: HIV-INFECTED WOMEN

The presenting signs and symptoms of PID generally do not differ significantly by HIV infection status,[81,82] although some studies have demonstrated an increased odds of fever, higher clinical severity scores, and higher likelihood of having a TOA among HIV-infected women.[83–85] Clinical severity has been found to correlate with immunosuppression among HIV-infected women with laparoscopically confirmed PID.[83]

Treatment of PID or TOA has been shown to be as effective in HIV-infected women as in uninfected women.[81,83,84,86] In a prospective study, the 12% clinical failure rate of outpatient therapy was not predicted by HIV serostatus.[81] Duration of hospitalization and antibiotic therapy also did not differ by HIV serostatus; however, among HIV-infected women, immunosuppressed patients required longer inpatient therapy and antibiotic regimens.[83]

SPECIAL POPULATIONS: POSTMENOPAUSAL WOMEN

Although rare, postmenopausal women can develop PID, presenting most commonly with lower abdominal pain and postmenopausal bleeding, as well as fever, nausea, and altered bowel habits; they are considerably more likely to have TOAs.[87,88] Among 20 postmenopausal women with TOAs in one case series, although only 20% of patients were febrile, 45% had elevated WBC counts, 55% had a palpable pelvic mass, and 90% had a TOA on surgical exploration.[89] In several small case series, pathologic analysis of the surgical specimens revealed a concurrent gynecologic malignancy (cervix, endometrium, or ovary) in 40% to 47% of the patients.[88–90] Based on these data, any postmenopausal woman with PID should be evaluated for the presence of a pelvic cancer.

SPECIAL POPULATIONS: INTRAUTERINE DEVICES

In the 1970s the Dalkon Shield intrauterine device (IUD) was associated with increased rates of PID, and led to significant concerns about the safety of IUDs in women at risk for STIs.[91] Modern IUDs, including the levonorgestrel IUD (Mirena) and the copper IUD (Paraguard), have not been associated with an increased risk of PID over the long term.[92] There does appear to be a slightly increased rate of PID in the 20 days after insertion: in one study the rate of PID during this time was 9.66 per 1000 women, in comparison with 1.38 per 1000 women thereafter.[93] A review of studies assessing PID after IUD insertion in the presence of gonococcal or chlamydial cervicitis showed an increased, but overall low risk (0%–5%).[94] Recent studies suggest that screening for gonorrhea and chlamydia at the time of insertion, as opposed to requiring a negative test before the procedure, does not significantly increase adverse sequelae.[95] There does not appear to be any difference in the risk for PID between hormone-containing and copper IUDs.[96] The presence of an IUD at the time of diagnosis of acute PID does not alter the management, and empiric removal of the IUD is not indicated.[67,97]

SEQUELAE

Women with PID have an increased risk of ectopic pregnancy, infertility, and chronic pelvic pain caused by tubal scarring and damage from inflammation. In the PEACH trial, 36% of participants reported chronic pelvic pain; women with 2 or more episodes of PID were at highest risk.[98] In a cohort study of women with laparoscopically confirmed salpingitis in Sweden, followed for a mean of 94 months, the infertility rate was 16%, 67% of which was attributable to tubal factor infertility, compared with an infertility rate of 2.7% in women without salpingitis. Of women who became pregnant, 9% of women with salpingitis had an ectopic pregnancy, compared with 1.9% of control women.[21] The risk of infertility increased with severity of salpingitis and number of episodes of PID. Chlamydial cervicitis also increases the risk of ectopic pregnancy with repeat infections; women with 3 or more episodes had 4.5 times increased odds of PID.[21]

In the PEACH trial, upper genital tract detection of gonorrhea, chlamydia, or endometritis was sufficient to confirm the diagnosis of PID. However, there were no differences in reproductive health outcomes between women with and without endometritis or upper genital tract infection.[42] A more recent study of women with lower genital tract infection but no PID by clinical criteria used a permissive definition of endometritis (1 plasma cell per high-power field) and showed a 40% decrease in pregnancy rates among women with endometritis (or subclinical PID).[44] The differences in these analyses may be due to a slightly higher rate of C trachomatis infection in the latter study.

PREVENTION

As gonorrhea and chlamydia contribute more than half to three-quarters of PID, screening for and treating these infections should decrease the incidence and sequelae. Four randomized trials have examined whether this strategy is effective. The earliest was conducted between 1990 and 1992 in Seattle, Washington. More than 1000 women in a managed care organization were randomized to receive an invitation for chlamydia screening, then followed for a year and compared with approximately 1600 women receiving standard care. Although only 64% of the intervention group were screened, during the 12-month follow-up there were 9 PID cases in the screening group and 33 in the control group (relative risk 0.44, 95% confidence interval 0.2–0.9).[99] A second study used cluster randomization to randomize students at 17 high schools to receive the offer of chlamydia screening, then followed them for PID over 12 months. At 1 year the PID incidence was 2.1% in the screening group (of whom 48% were screened) and 4.2% in the control group.[100] Most recently, the Prevention Of Pelvic Infections (POPI) trial in England enrolled sexually active women younger than 27 years and randomized them to early versus delayed screening for chlamydia. The early screening group had a chlamydia prevalence of 5.4%, and 15 of 1191 (1.3%) developed PID over the course of the study. In the delayed group, 5.9% had chlamydia detected on their enrollment swab when it was tested a year later. During that time, 23 of 1186 (1.9%) in this group developed PID. The relative risk for PID in those with early screening was not significant (0.65; 95% confidence interval 0.34–1.22),[32] but the study was under-powered given the low rate of PID.

SUMMARY

PID is associated with significant reproductive morbidity, which appears to be reduced with prompt, proactive treatment of cervicitis and lower genital tract infections. It is a clinical diagnosis, and providers should maintain a high index of suspicion when presented with a woman of reproductive age complaining of abdominal and pelvic pain. STIs are commonly associated with PID, but vaginal anaerobes also seem to be involved, and antibiotic coverage for these pathogens should be considered when treating women with severe symptoms or pelvic abscesses.

REFERENCES

1. Rein DB, Kassler WJ, Irwin KL, et al. Direct medical cost of pelvic inflammatory disease and its sequelae: decreasing, but still substantial. Obstet Gynecol 2000;95(3):397–402.
2. Bender N, Herrmann B, Andersen B, et al. Chlamydia infection, pelvic inflammatory disease, ectopic pregnancy and infertility: cross-national study. Sex Transm Infect 2011;87(7):601–8.
3. Paik CK, Waetjen LE, Xing G, et al. Hospitalizations for pelvic inflammatory disease and tuboovarian abscess. Obstet Gynecol 2006;107(3):611–6.
4. Sutton MY, Sternberg M, Zaidi A, et al. Trends in pelvic inflammatory disease hospital discharges and ambulatory visits, United States, 1985-2001. Sex Transm Dis 2005;32(12):778–84.
5. Owusu-Edusei K Jr, Bohm MK, Chesson HW, et al. Chlamydia screening and pelvic inflammatory disease: insights from exploratory time-series analyses. Am J Prev Med 2010;38(6):652–7.
6. Bohm MK, Newman L, Satterwhite CL, et al. Pelvic inflammatory disease among privately insured women, United States, 2001-2005. Sex Transm Dis 2010;37(3):131–6.
7. Ness RB, Soper DE, Holley RL, et al. Hormonal and barrier contraception and risk of upper genital tract disease in the PID Evaluation and Clinical Health (PEACH) study. Am J Obstet Gynecol 2001;185(1):121–7.
8. Ness RB, Soper DE, Holley RL, et al. Douching and endometritis: results from the PID Evaluation and Clinical Health (PEACH) study. Sex Transm Dis 2001;28(4):240–5.
9. Simms I, Stephenson JM, Mallinson H, et al. Risk factors associated with pelvic inflammatory disease. Sex Transm Infect 2006;82(6):452–7.
10. Scholes D, Daling JR, Stergachis A, et al. Vaginal douching as a risk factor for acute pelvic inflammatory disease. Obstet Gynecol 1993;81(4):601–6.
11. Wolner-Hanssen P, Eschenbach DA, Paavonen J, et al. Association between vaginal douching and acute pelvic inflammatory disease. JAMA 1990;263(14):1936–41.
12. Kimani J, Maclean IW, Bwayo JJ, et al. Risk factors for Chlamydia trachomatis pelvic inflammatory disease among sex workers in Nairobi, Kenya. J Infect Dis 1996;173(6):1437–44.
13. Ness RB, Keder LM, Soper DE, et al. Oral contraception and the recognition of endometritis. Am J Obstet Gynecol 1997;176(3):580–5.
14. Wolner-Hanssen P, Svensson L, Mardh PA, et al. Laparoscopic findings and contraceptive use in women with signs and symptoms suggestive of acute salpingitis. Obstet Gynecol 1985;66(2):233–8.
15. Taylor BD, Darville T, Haggerty CL. Does bacterial vaginosis cause pelvic inflammatory disease? Sex Transm Dis 2013;40(2):117–22.
16. Ness RB, Hillier SL, Kip KE, et al. Bacterial vaginosis and risk of pelvic inflammatory disease. Obstet Gynecol 2004;104(4):761–9.
17. Eschenbach DA, Buchanan TM, Pollock HM, et al. Polymicrobial etiology of acute pelvic inflammatory disease. N Engl J Med 1975;293(4):166–71.
18. Sweet RL. Pelvic inflammatory disease. Sex Transm Dis 1986;13(Suppl 3):192–8.

19. Taylor BD, Ness RB, Darville T, et al. Microbial correlates of delayed care for pelvic inflammatory disease. Sex Transm Dis 2011;38(5):434–8.
20. Haggerty CL, Totten PA, Astete SG, et al. *Mycoplasma genitalium* among women with nongonococcal, nonchlamydial pelvic inflammatory disease. Infect Dis Obstet Gynecol 2006;2006:30184.
21. Westrom L, Joesoef R, Reynolds G, et al. Pelvic inflammatory disease and fertility. A cohort study of 1,844 women with laparoscopically verified disease and 657 control women with normal laparoscopic results. Sex Transm Dis 1992;19(4):185–92.
22. Heinonen PK, Miettinen A. Laparoscopic study on the microbiology and severity of acute pelvic inflammatory disease. Eur J Obstet Gynecol Reprod Biol 1994; 57(2):85–9.
23. Hillier SL, Kiviat NB, Hawes SE, et al. Role of bacterial vaginosis-associated microorganisms in endometritis. Am J Obstet Gynecol 1996;175(2):435–41.
24. Taylor-Robinson D, Jensen JS, Svenstrup H, et al. Difficulties experienced in defining the microbial cause of pelvic inflammatory disease. Int J STD AIDS 2012;23(1):18–24.
25. Bjartling C, Osser S, Persson K. *Mycoplasma genitalium* in cervicitis and pelvic inflammatory disease among women at a gynecologic outpatient service. Am J Obstet Gynecol 2012;206(6):476.e1–8.
26. Cohen CR, Manhart LE, Bukusi EA, et al. Association between *Mycoplasma genitalium* and acute endometritis. Lancet 2002;359(9308):765–6.
27. Soper DE, Brockwell NJ, Dalton HP, et al. Observations concerning the microbial etiology of acute salpingitis. Am J Obstet Gynecol 1994;170(4):1008–14 [discussion: 14–7].
28. Wasserheit JN, Bell TA, Kiviat NB, et al. Microbial causes of proven pelvic inflammatory disease and efficacy of clindamycin and tobramycin. Ann Intern Med 1986;104(2):187–93.
29. Hebb JK, Cohen CR, Astete SG, et al. Detection of novel organisms associated with salpingitis, by use of 16S rRNA polymerase chain reaction. J Infect Dis 2004;190(12):2109–20.
30. Herzog SA, Althaus CL, Heijne JC, et al. Timing of progression from *Chlamydia trachomatis* infection to pelvic inflammatory disease: a mathematical modelling study. BMC Infect Dis 2012;12:187.
31. Morre SA, van den Brule AJ, Rozendaal L, et al. The natural course of asymptomatic *Chlamydia trachomatis* infections: 45% clearance and no development of clinical PID after one-year follow-up. Int J STD AIDS 2002; 13(Suppl 2):12–8.
32. Oakeshott P, Kerry S, Aghaizu A, et al. Randomised controlled trial of screening for *Chlamydia trachomatis* to prevent pelvic inflammatory disease: the POPI (Prevention of Pelvic Infection) trial. BMJ 2010;340:c1642.
33. Katz DF. Human cervical mucus: research update. Am J Obstet Gynecol 1991; 165(6 Pt 2):1984–6.
34. Kunz G, Beil D, Deininger H, et al. The dynamics of rapid sperm transport through the female genital tract: evidence from vaginal sonography of uterine peristalsis and hysterosalpingoscintigraphy. Hum Reprod 1996;11(3):627–32.
35. Darville T, Hiltke TJ. Pathogenesis of genital tract disease due to *Chlamydia trachomatis*. J Infect Dis 2010;201(Suppl 2):S114–25.
36. Patton DL, Kuo CC. Histopathology of *Chlamydia trachomatis* salpingitis after primary and repeated reinfections in the monkey subcutaneous pocket model. J Reprod Fertil 1989;85(2):647–56.

37. Van Voorhis WC, Barrett LK, Sweeney YT, et al. Repeated *Chlamydia trachomatis* infection of *Macaca nemestrina* fallopian tubes produces a th1-like cytokine response associated with fibrosis and scarring. Infect Immun 1997;65(6): 2175–82.

38. Peeling RW, Kimani J, Plummer F, et al. Antibody to chlamydial hsp60 predicts an increased risk for chlamydial pelvic inflammatory disease. J Infect Dis 1997; 175(5):1153–8.

39. Toye B, Laferriere C, Claman P, et al. Association between antibody to the chlamydial heat-shock protein and tubal infertility. J Infect Dis 1993;168(5):1236–40.

40. Ness RB, Soper DE, Richter HE, et al. Chlamydia antibodies, chlamydia heat shock protein, and adverse sequelae after pelvic inflammatory disease: the PID Evaluation and Clinical Health (PEACH) study. Sex Transm Dis 2008; 35(2):129–35.

41. Kiviat NB, Wolner-Hanssen P, Eschenbach DA, et al. Endometrial histopathology in patients with culture-proved upper genital tract infection and laparoscopically diagnosed acute salpingitis. Am J Surg Pathol 1990;14(2):167–75.

42. Haggerty CL, Ness RB, Amortegui A, et al. Endometritis does not predict reproductive morbidity after pelvic inflammatory disease. Am J Obstet Gynecol 2003; 188(1):141–8.

43. Achilles SL, Amortegui AJ, Wiesenfeld HC. Endometrial plasma cells: do they indicate subclinical pelvic inflammatory disease? Sex Transm Dis 2005;32(3): 185–8.

44. Wiesenfeld HC, Hillier SL, Meyn LA, et al. Subclinical pelvic inflammatory disease and infertility. Obstet Gynecol 2012;120(1):37–43.

45. Jacobson L. Differential diagnosis of acute pelvic inflammatory disease. Am J Obstet Gynecol 1980;138(7 Pt 2):1006–11.

46. Short VL, Totten PA, Ness RB, et al. Clinical presentation of *Mycoplasma genitalium* infection versus *Neisseria gonorrhoeae* infection among women with pelvic inflammatory disease. Clin Infect Dis 2009;48(1):41–7.

47. Jacobson L, Westrom L. Objectivized diagnosis of acute pelvic inflammatory disease. Diagnostic and prognostic value of routine laparoscopy. Am J Obstet Gynecol 1969;105(7):1088–98.

48. Simms I, Eastick K, Mallinson H, et al. Associations between *Mycoplasma genitalium*, *Chlamydia trachomatis*, and pelvic inflammatory disease. Sex Transm Infect 2003;79(2):154–6.

49. Eckert LO, Hawes SE, Wolner-Hanssen PK, et al. Endometritis: the clinical-pathologic syndrome. Am J Obstet Gynecol 2002;186(4):690–5.

50. Paavonen J, Kiviat N, Brunham RC, et al. Prevalence and manifestations of endometritis among women with cervicitis. Am J Obstet Gynecol 1985;152(3):280–6.

51. Kahn JG, Walker CK, Washington AE, et al. Diagnosing pelvic inflammatory disease. A comprehensive analysis and considerations for developing a new model. JAMA 1991;266(18):2594–604.

52. Peipert JF, Ness RB, Blume J, et al. Clinical predictors of endometritis in women with symptoms and signs of pelvic inflammatory disease. Am J Obstet Gynecol 2001;184(5):856–63 [discussion: 63–4].

53. Yudin MH, Hillier SL, Wiesenfeld HC, et al. Vaginal polymorphonuclear leukocytes and bacterial vaginosis as markers for histologic endometritis among women without symptoms of pelvic inflammatory disease. Am J Obstet Gynecol 2003;188(2):318–23.

54. Peipert JF, Boardman L, Hogan JW, et al. Laboratory evaluation of acute upper genital tract infection. Obstet Gynecol 1996;87(5 Pt 1):730–6.

55. Cacciatore B, Leminen A, Ingman-Friberg S, et al. Transvaginal sonographic findings in ambulatory patients with suspected pelvic inflammatory disease. Obstet Gynecol 1992;80(6):912–6.
56. Timor-Tritsch IE, Lerner JP, Monteagudo A, et al. Transvaginal sonographic markers of tubal inflammatory disease. Ultrasound Obstet Gynecol 1998; 12(1):56–66.
57. Molander P, Finne P, Sjoberg J, et al. Observer agreement with laparoscopic diagnosis of pelvic inflammatory disease using photographs. Obstet Gynecol 2003;101(5 Pt 1):875–80.
58. Tukeva TA, Aronen HJ, Karjalainen PT, et al. MR imaging in pelvic inflammatory disease: comparison with laparoscopy and us. Radiology 1999;210(1): 209–16.
59. Wolner-Hanssen P, Paavonen J, Kiviat N, et al. Outpatient treatment of pelvic inflammatory disease with cefoxitin and doxycycline. Obstet Gynecol 1988;71(4): 595–600.
60. Arredondo JL, Diaz V, Gaitan H, et al. Oral clindamycin and ciprofloxacin versus intramuscular ceftriaxone and oral doxycycline in the treatment of mild-to-moderate pelvic inflammatory disease in outpatients. Clin Infect Dis 1997; 24(2):170–8.
61. Ness RB, Soper DE, Holley RL, et al. Effectiveness of inpatient and outpatient treatment strategies for women with pelvic inflammatory disease: results from the Pelvic Inflammatory Disease Evaluation and Clinical Health (PEACH) randomized trial. Am J Obstet Gynecol 2002;186(5):929–37.
62. Ness RB, Trautmann G, Richter HE, et al. Effectiveness of treatment strategies of some women with pelvic inflammatory disease: a randomized trial. Obstet Gynecol 2005;106(3):573–80.
63. Dunbar-Jacob J, Sereika SM, Foley SM, et al. Adherence to oral therapies in pelvic inflammatory disease. J Womens Health (Larchmt) 2004;13(3):285–91.
64. Augenbraun MH, McCormack WH. Pelvic inflammatory disease: an ongoing epidemic. Hosp Pract (1995) 1995;30(9):61–6.
65. Katz BP, Zwickl BW, Caine VA, et al. Compliance with antibiotic therapy for Chlamydia trachomatis and Neisseria gonorrhoeae. Sex Transm Dis 1992; 19(6):351–4.
66. Hemsell DL, Little BB, Faro S, et al. Comparison of three regimens recommended by the centers for disease control and prevention for the treatment of women hospitalized with acute pelvic inflammatory disease. Clin Infect Dis 1994;19(4):720–7.
67. Workowski KA, Berman S. Sexually transmitted diseases treatment guidelines, 2010. MMWR Recomm Rep 2010;59(RR-12):1–110.
68. Workowski KA, Berman SM. Sexually transmitted diseases treatment guidelines, 2006. MMWR Recomm Rep 2006;55(RR-11):1–94.
69. Katz AR, Lee MV, Wasserman GM. Sexually transmitted disease (STD) update: a review of the CDC 2010 STD treatment guidelines and epidemiologic trends of common STDs in Hawai'i. Hawaii J Med Public Health 2012;71(3):68–73.
70. Bevan CD, Ridgway GL, Rothermel CD. Efficacy and safety of azithromycin as monotherapy or combined with metronidazole compared with two standard multidrug regimens for the treatment of acute pelvic inflammatory disease. J Int Med Res 2003;31(1):45–54.
71. Savaris RF, Teixeira LM, Torres TG, et al. Comparing ceftriaxone plus azithromycin or doxycycline for pelvic inflammatory disease: a randomized controlled trial. Obstet Gynecol 2007;110(1):53–60.

72. Haggerty CL, Totten PA, Astete SG, et al. Failure of cefoxitin and doxycycline to eradicate endometrial *Mycoplasma genitalium* and the consequence for clinical cure of pelvic inflammatory disease. Sex Transm Infect 2008;84(5):338–42.

73. Manhart LE, Broad JM, Golden MR. *Mycoplasma genitalium*: should we treat and how? Clin Infect Dis 2011;53(Suppl 3):S129–42.

74. Haggerty CL, Hillier SL, Bass DC, et al. Bacterial vaginosis and anaerobic bacteria are associated with endometritis. Clin Infect Dis 2004;39(7):990–5.

75. Swidsinski A, Verstraelen H, Loening-Baucke V, et al. Presence of a polymicrobial endometrial biofilm in patients with bacterial vaginosis. PLoS One 2013; 8(1):e53997.

76. Walker CK, Workowski KA, Washington AE, et al. Anaerobes in pelvic inflammatory disease: implications for the centers for disease control and prevention's guidelines for treatment of sexually transmitted diseases. Clin Infect Dis 1999; 28(Suppl 1):S29–36.

77. Landers DV, Sweet RL. Tubo-ovarian abscess: contemporary approach to management. Rev Infect Dis 1983;5(5):876–84.

78. Reed SD, Landers DV, Sweet RL. Antibiotic treatment of tuboovarian abscess: comparison of broad-spectrum beta-lactam agents versus clindamycin-containing regimens. Am J Obstet Gynecol 1991;164(6 Pt 1):1556–61 [discussion: 61–2].

79. Gjelland K, Ekerhovd E, Granberg S. Transvaginal ultrasound-guided aspiration for treatment of tubo-ovarian abscess: a study of 302 cases. Am J Obstet Gynecol 2005;193(4):1323–30.

80. Goharkhay N, Verma U, Maggiorotto F. Comparison of CT- or ultrasound-guided drainage with concomitant intravenous antibiotics vs. intravenous antibiotics alone in the management of tubo-ovarian abscesses. Ultrasound Obstet Gynecol 2007;29(1):65–9.

81. Irwin KL, Moorman AC, O'Sullivan MJ, et al. Influence of human immunodeficiency virus infection on pelvic inflammatory disease. Obstet Gynecol 2000; 95(4):525–34.

82. Korn AP, Landers DV, Green JR, et al. Pelvic inflammatory disease in human immunodeficiency virus-infected women. Obstet Gynecol 1993;82(5):765–8.

83. Cohen CR, Sinei S, Reilly M, et al. Effect of human immunodeficiency virus type 1 infection upon acute salpingitis: a laparoscopic study. J Infect Dis 1998; 178(5):1352–8.

84. Kamenga MC, De Cock KM, St Louis ME, et al. The impact of human immunodeficiency virus infection on pelvic inflammatory disease: a case-control study in Abidjan, Ivory Coast. Am J Obstet Gynecol 1995;172(3):919–25.

85. Mugo NR, Kiehlbauch JA, Nguti R, et al. Effect of human immunodeficiency virus-1 infection on treatment outcome of acute salpingitis. Obstet Gynecol 2006;107(4):807–12.

86. Bukusi EA, Cohen CR, Stevens CE, et al. Effects of human immunodeficiency virus 1 infection on microbial origins of pelvic inflammatory disease and on efficacy of ambulatory oral therapy. Am J Obstet Gynecol 1999;181(6):1374–81.

87. Heaton FC, Ledger WJ. Postmenopausal tuboovarian abscess. Obstet Gynecol 1976;47(1):90–4.

88. Protopapas AG, Diakomanolis ES, Milingos SD, et al. Tubo-ovarian abscesses in postmenopausal women: gynecological malignancy until proven otherwise? Eur J Obstet Gynecol Reprod Biol 2004;114(2):203–9.

89. Lipscomb GH, Ling FW. Tubo-ovarian abscess in postmenopausal patients. South Med J 1992;85(7):696–9.

90. Hoffman M, Molpus K, Roberts WS, et al. Tuboovarian abscess in postmeno-pausal women. J Reprod Med 1990;35(5):525–8.
91. Gareen IF, Greenland S, Morgenstern H. Intrauterine devices and pelvic inflam-matory disease: meta-analyses of published studies, 1974-1990. Epidemiology 2000;11(5):589–97.
92. Feldblum PJ, Caraway J, Bahamondes L, et al. Randomized assignment to cop-per IUD or depot-medroxyprogesterone acetate: feasibility of enrollment, contin-uation and disease ascertainment. Contraception 2005;72(3):187–91.
93. Farley TM, Rosenberg MJ, Rowe PJ, et al. Intrauterine devices and pelvic inflam-matory disease: an international perspective. Lancet 1992;339(8796):785–8.
94. Mohllajee AP, Curtis KM, Peterson HB. Does insertion and use of an intrauterine de-vice increase the risk of pelvic inflammatory disease among women with sexually transmitted infection? A systematic review. Contraception 2006;73(2):145–53.
95. Sufrin CB, Postlethwaite D, Armstrong MA, et al. *Neisseria gonorrhoeae* and *Chlamydia trachomatis* screening at intrauterine device insertion and pelvic in-flammatory disease. Obstet Gynecol 2012;120(6):1314–21.
96. Sivin I, Stern J, Diaz J, et al. Two years of intrauterine contraception with levonor-gestrel and with copper: a randomized comparison of the TCU 380ag and levo-norgestrel 20 mcg/day devices. Contraception 1987;35(3):245–55.
97. Soderberg G, Lindgren S. Influence of an intrauterine device on the course of an acute salpingitis. Contraception 1981;24(2):137–43.
98. Haggerty CL, Peipert JF, Weitzen S, et al. Predictors of chronic pelvic pain in an urban population of women with symptoms and signs of pelvic inflammatory dis-ease. Sex Transm Dis 2005;32(5):293–9.
99. Scholes D, Stergachis A, Heidrich FE, et al. Prevention of pelvic inflammatory disease by screening for cervical chlamydial infection. N Engl J Med 1996;334(21):1362–6.
100. Ostergaard L, Andersen B, Moller JK, et al. Home sampling versus conventional swab sampling for screening of *Chlamydia trachomatis* in women: a cluster-randomized 1-year follow-up study. Clin Infect Dis 2000;31(4):951–7.
101. Marrazzo JM, Martin DH. Management of women with cervicitis. Clin Infect Dis 2007;44(Suppl 3):S102–10.
102. Paavonen J, Aine R, Teisala K, et al. Comparison of endometrial biopsy and peri-toneal fluid cytologic testing with laparoscopy in the diagnosis of acute pelvic inflammatory disease. Am J Obstet Gynecol 1985;151(5):645–50.
103. Walker CK, Landers DV, Ohm-Smith MJ, et al. Comparison of cefotetan plus doxycycline with cefoxitin plus doxycycline in the inpatient treatment of acute salpingitis. Sex Transm Dis 1991;18(2):119–23.
104. Comparative evaluation of clindamycin/gentamicin and cefoxitin/doxycycline for treatment of pelvic inflammatory disease: a multi-center trial. The European Study Group. Acta Obstet Gynecol Scand 1992;71(2):129–34.
105. McGregor JA, Crombleholme WR, Newton E, et al. Randomized comparison of ampicillin-sulbactam to cefoxitin and doxycycline or clindamycin and genta-micin in the treatment of pelvic inflammatory disease or endometritis. Obstet Gynecol 1994;83(6):998–1004.
106. Walters MD, Gibbs RS. A randomized comparison of gentamicin-clindamycin and cefoxitin-doxycycline in the treatment of acute pelvic inflammatory disease. Obstet Gynecol 1990;75(5):867–72.
107. Piyadigamage A, Wilson J. Improvement in the clinical cure rate of outpatient management of pelvic inflammatory disease following a change in therapy. Sex Transm Infect 2005;81(3):233–5.

Sexual Transmission of Viral Hepatitis

Linda Gorgos, MD, MSc

KEYWORDS

- Viral hepatitis • Hepatitis A • Hepatitis B • Hepatitis C • Sexual transmission
- Prevention

KEY POINTS

- Epidemiologic and molecular data support the role of sexual transmission in outbreaks and regional transmission of hepatitis A among men with male sex partners (MSM). There is little evidence to suggest that sexual contact plays a significant role as a mode of transmission among heterosexual partners. Hepatitis A vaccine is the most effective means of prevention among at-risk adults.
- Hepatitis B (HBV) is efficiently transmitted through sexual contact between men and women and between MSM. Identification and vaccination of adults at risk for HBV acquisition through sexual contact is a key strategy to reduce new HBV infections among at-risk adults. High levels of coverage for hepatitis B immunization in at-risk adults, including populations attending sexually transmitted disease clinics, MSM, and MSM infected with the human immunodeficiency virus (HIV), remain elusive, and clinicians should be vigilant in recommending vaccination to such persons.
- Transmission of hepatitis C virus (HCV) through heterosexual contact seems to be inefficient, with previous studies showing transmission among long-term monogamous heterosexual partners occurring in less than 1% of couples per year. Heterosexual transmission of HCV may occur more efficiently in the presence of other biological and behavioral risks, including HIV coinfection, higher-risk sexual practices, and in the presence of other sexually transmitted infections (STIs).
- Hepatitis C has emerged as an STI among MSM, primarily among MSM who are HIV-infected. Several factors have been linked to HCV transmission among MSM, including HIV coinfection; participation in sexual practices that result in mucosal damage or result in exposure to blood; presence of STIs, particularly ulcerative STIs; multiple/casual sex partners; and unprotected anal intercourse.

INTRODUCTION

Although hepatitis B has long been recognized as a sexually transmitted infection (STI), the role of sexual contact in the transmission of hepatitis A and hepatitis C has been less clear. Ongoing epidemiologic studies and the more recent availability

Potential Conflicts of Interest: None.
Special Immunology Associates, El Rio Health Center, 1701 West St Mary's Road, Suite 160, Tucson, AZ 85745, USA
E-mail address: lindag@elrio.org

Infect Dis Clin N Am 27 (2013) 811–836
http://dx.doi.org/10.1016/j.idc.2013.08.002
0891-5520/13/$ – see front matter © 2013 Elsevier Inc. All rights reserved.

of molecular methods to investigate transmission patterns of viral hepatitis have broadened the understanding of hepatitis A and C as STIs among at-risk adults. This review focuses on previous knowledge and current developments in the understanding of hepatitis A, B, and C as STIs and discusses means of preventing infection.

Methods

A systematic search of the literature on sexual transmission of viral hepatitis was conducted using PubMed (National Library of Medicine) in February, 2013. Medical Subject Heading (MeSH) terms, MeSH subheadings, and key words used included "hepatitis A," "hepatitis B," "hepatitis C," "hepatitis D," "epidemiology," "men who have sex with men," "homosexuality, male," "MSM," "transmission," "sexual transmission," and "prevention and control."

HEPATITIS A

Hepatitis A virus (HAV) is a small unenveloped RNA virus. The virus replicates in the liver, is excreted into bile, and is shed in the stool, resulting in spread by the fecal-oral route. Concentration of virus in the stool is highest in the 2 weeks before onset of clinical illness with jaundice or increase in liver enzyme levels, and declines after jaundice appears.[1] Transmission can occur through contaminated food or water and through person-to-person transmission among close contacts in household, institutional, and child care settings. Small children may play an important role in transmission in household and close contact settings.[2–6]

Sexual contact and certain sexual practices may also result in contact to and transmission of HAV. Several studies have examined HAV seroprevalence in at-risk adults, primarily among persons attending sexually transmitted disease (STD) clinics or other high-risk groups (street youth, drug users). Reported HAV seroprevalence in the STD clinic setting has ranged from 29% to 60%, with most studies showing a seroprevalence in the 30% to 40% range.[7–14] Factors reported in association with HAV seroprevalence among STD clinic attendees include the following: increasing age,[7,8] ethnicity,[7] lower levels of education attainment,[8] increasing numbers of sex partners,[8,10] current genital herpes,[8] and syphilis.[8,13] A Canadian study compared HAV seroprevalence among female student nurses (13%) and blood donors (11% in men, 14% in women) with STD clinic attendees (37% in men, 35% in women).[10] Few have compared seroprevalence among STD clinic attendees to age-matched and sex-matched general population controls or have controlled for potential confounding factors. In a prospective cohort of MSM and heterosexual men, the annual incidence of hepatitis A in susceptible MSM was 22%, whereas no heterosexual men acquired hepatitis A.[15] There is little evidence to support heterosexual contact as a significant mode of HAV transmission.

Many studies have investigated HAV seroprevalence among men reporting male sex partners (MSM). These studies have included STD clinic–based samples, community-based convenience samples, and street youth. In 2 cohorts of MSM in Australia, HAV seroprevalence was 68% in HIV-infected MSM and 69% in HIV-negative MSM.[16] Young MSM tested in California had an HAV seroprevalence of 28%, with 3.3% showing evidence of recent HAV infections. Predictors of prevalent infection included Latino ethnicity, report of 50 or more lifetime sex partners, and less than high school education; recent infection was associated with less than a high school education, insertive anal intercourse, and sharing needles without cleaning them.[17] HAV prevalence in a sample of MSM and injection drug users (IDU) followed in 2 prospective cohort studies in the United States was compared with a sample of blood donors. Hepatitis A prevalence was 66% in IDU, 32% in MSM, and 14% in blood donors. Age-adjusted prevalence among MSM (28%) was similar to the US general population age-adjusted seroprevalence (31%).[18] Most STD clinic–based samples have shown no difference in HAV seroprevalence in MSM versus men reporting female sex partners[7–10,12,14]; however, not all studies have controlled for other potential confounders, including age, ethnicity, country of birth, drug use, and socioeconomic status. In a prospective cohort of MSM and men with female sex partners followed for 9 months and 6 months, respectively, seroprevalence was 30% in MSM and 12% in heterosexual men ($P<.01$).[15] For MSM enrolled in a hepatitis vaccine trial and followed for 24 months, 14% acquired new HAV infection, and incident HAV was associated with the number of sex partners in the preceding 6 months.[19]

Multiple outbreaks of HAV among MSM have been reported in North America, Europe, Australia, and Japan.[20–34] A commonly reported risk for HAV acquisition among MSM is casual or anonymous sex partners or sex in venues where contact with casual partners is more common.[7,21,22,24,27] Several investigations examined the potential role of specific sexual practices in HAV acquisition. Although some have shown no link between specific sexual practices among MSM and HAV seroprevalence,[7,9,26] others have shown an association with oral-anal sex,[12,21,25] digital-anal contact,[21] and insertive anal intercourse.[17,35] In a prospective cohort of MSM, incident HAV infection was associated with frequent oral-anal contact, as detailed in diaries of sexual behavior.[15]

The use of molecular epidemiologic methods has documented the circulation of specific HAV strains within populations of MSM. A prospective study of community-acquired HAV cases reported in Amsterdam reported clustering of genotypes within separate transmission circles. Clusters of a specific genotype occurred within networks of MSM cases, whereas separate and distinct genotypes were seen among cases linked to children returning from HAV-endemic countries and their contacts.[36] Transmission among travelers was sporadic, with a seasonal pattern associated with the summer holidays. The MSM clusters were larger and persisted over longer periods, suggesting ongoing endemic spread within the local MSM community.[37] A collaborative study in Denmark, Germany, the Netherlands, Norway, Spain, and the United Kingdom[38] examined genetic sequences of HAV isolates collected from 1997 to 2005. Most strains found among MSM from the different countries formed a closely related cluster, whereas different HAV strains circulated among other risk groups in these countries during the same period. It appeared that specific strains were circulating exclusively among MSM over a long period across a wide geographic region, suggesting endemic HAV transmission among MSM. The epidemiologic and molecular data support the potential for sexual transmission of HAV among MSM. It is plausible that specific sexual practices (oral-anal contact, digital-anal contact, anal intercourse) may increase potential exposure to HAV, as can higher-risk partnerships (casual partners, higher number of partners, sexual contact within venues for casual sex).

Prevention of Hepatitis A

Immunization is the most effective means available to reduce hepatitis A infection among adults at risk through sexual exposure. Hepatitis A vaccines became available in 1995 and are highly immunogenic in adults. Nearly all adults (94%–100%) develop protective antibody levels 1 month after an initial dose, with a second dose of scheduled vaccine providing protective antibody in 100% of healthy adults.[39–41] Protective levels of HAV antibody persist in adults for more than 10 years, and modeling studies suggest that protection may last 25 years or more in adults.[39,42] Hepatitis A vaccine is immunogenic for adults with HIV infection, although adults with lower CD4 counts are less likely to develop protective levels of antibody.[43–47]

Immunization strategies for hepatitis A vary by country. Since licensure of hepatitis A vaccine in 1995 to 1996, the hepatitis A childhood immunization strategy in the United States was implemented incrementally, initially targeting children living in communities with the highest disease rates. In 2006, the US Advisory Committee on Immunization Practices (ACIP) expanded recommendations to include the routine vaccination of children older than 1 year in the United States.[39,48,49] Although younger birth cohorts in countries that have implemented routine childhood HAV immunization programs are likely to remain protected from HAV well in to adulthood, many adults may remain susceptible.

In 1996, ACIP advised that MSM receive hepatitis A vaccination. Current recommendations for hepatitis A vaccination in the United States and in Canada include MSM as a target group for vaccination.[39,50] Despite this recommendation, vaccine implementation in this group in the United States seems incomplete. Among MSM visiting an urban sexual health program in 1999 to 2000, 72% of MSM reported that they were eligible to receive both HAV and HBV vaccine based on having no history of previous vaccination or infection. Of those eligible for vaccine, 63% accepted a first dose.[51] Even in high-risk groups engaged in routine medical care, vaccination rates remain low. In a retrospective survey of HIV-infected MSM followed at 8 HIV clinics from 2004 to 2007,[52] only 29% who were HAV susceptible by serologic testing were subsequently vaccinated for hepatitis A. In annual convenience surveys of MSM across multiple US cities from 1999 to 2004,[53] vaccination rates against hepatitis A did increase from 21% to 48%. These studies highlight the challenges of reaching high-risk adult populations for vaccination.

HAV vaccines currently licensed in the United States are the single-antigen vaccines HAVRIX (GlaxoSmithKline, Rixensart, Belgium) and VAQTA (Merck, Whitehouse Station, NJ) and the combination vaccine TWINRIX (containing both HAV and HBV antigens; GlaxoSmithKline). Dosage and schedules for HAV vaccine administration in adults and adolescents are shown in **Table 1**. In addition to vaccination, MSM should also be counseled about the potential for sexual transmission of HAV and sexual behaviors that may increase the risk for sexually acquired HAV (multiple partners, casual/anonymous partners, oral-anal contact, digital-anal contact). Barrier methods,

Table 1
Recommended dose and schedule for hepatitis A vaccines

Vaccine	Age (y)	Dose	Volume (mL)	No. of Doses	Dose Schedule (mo)[a]
HAVRIX[b]	1–18	720 (ELU)	0.5	2	0, 6–12
	>18	1440 (ELU)	1.0	2	0, 6–12
VAQTA[c]	1–18	25 (U)	0.5	2	0, 6–18
	>18	50 (U)	1.0	2	0, 6–18
TWINRIX[d]	≥18	720 (ELU)/20 μg	1.0	3	0, 1, 6

Abbreviations: ELU, enzyme-linked immunosorbent assay units; U, units.
    [a] 0 month represents timing of the initial dose; subsequent numbers represent months after the initial dose.
    [b] Hepatitis A vaccine, inactivated, GlaxoSmithKline (Rixensart, Belgium); this vaccine is also licensed for a 3-dose series in children aged 2–18 years, with 360-ELU, 0.5-mL doses at 0, 1, and 6–12 months.
    [c] Hepatitis A vaccine, inactivated, Merck (Whitehouse Station, NJ).
    [d] Combined hepatitis A and hepatitis B vaccine, GlaxoSmithKline (Rixensart, Belgium).
    Data from Fiore AE, Wasley A, Bell BP. Prevention of hepatitis A through active or passive immunization: recommendations of the Advisory Committee on Immunization Practices (ACIP). MMWR Recomm Rep 2006;55(RR-7):1–23.

including condoms, gloves, and dental dams, can be used to reduce potential for contact with HAV.

HEPATITIS B

Hepatitis B virus (HBV) is an enveloped, double-stranded DNA virus that can cause both acute and chronic infection. Potential consequences of chronic HBV infection include chronic liver disease, cirrhosis, and hepatocellular carcinoma. It is estimated that more than 2 billion people worldwide have been infected with hepatitis B, with approximately 360 million persons chronically infected.[54] Mathematical models for 2000 estimated that 620,000 persons died worldwide from HBV-related causes, including 580,000 (94%) from chronic infection-related cirrhosis and hepatocellular carcinoma and 40,000 (6%) from acute hepatitis B.[55] Transmission of HBV occurs through percutaneous or mucosal contact with infected blood or infectious body fluids. Modes of percutaneous transmission include transfusion of infected blood or blood products; receipt of HBV-infected organs or tissues; contact via injection drug use; occupational exposure in health care workers; and exposure in health care settings with inadequate infection control measures. HBV can be transmitted vertically from mother to child or from person to person through close (nonsexual) interpersonal contact with infected individuals (namely, among household contacts of persons with HBV infection).

Hepatitis B is also efficiently transmitted via sexual contact with infected individuals, an observation supported by epidemiologic and biological data. Hepatitis B surface antigen (HBsAg) or HBV DNA has been detected in body fluids and mucosal surfaces of infected individuals, including semen,[56–58] menstrual blood/vaginal discharge,[56,59] saliva,[58] feces,[60,61] anal canal and rectal mucosa,[61] and rectal mucosal lesions.[61] Animal models have shown the infectiousness of human semen by intravaginal instillation[62] or inoculation,[62,63] and case reports of HBV infection transmitted by artificial insemination support the role of semen in transmission of HBV in humans.[57]

A US investigation of household contacts to acute HBV cases in 1977 found that 23% of susceptible spouses or sexual contacts of acute HBV cases developed hepatitis B infection during the 6-month follow-up period, whereas no new infections were found in parents, siblings, and other domestic contacts.[64] Among persons exposed to a spouse with acute HBV infection who were randomized to the placebo arm of a prophylaxis trial, 27% developed symptomatic hepatitis B, whereas another 15% developed subclinical hepatitis B.[65]

Multiple studies have reported high levels of past or present HBV infection among groups believed to be at higher risk via sexual exposure, including persons attending STD clinics, commercial sex workers (CSW), and MSM. HBV seroprevalence reported among CSW has ranged from 8% to 67%,[66–72] with a higher HBV prevalence among CSW relative to controls.[68,70] HBV acquisition was common, with a mean annual incidence of 4.7% among Peruvian CSW,[69] similar to a reported 10% acquisition over 2 years in another study of CSW.[67] Reported risk factors associated with prevalent HBV infection in this group were syphilis,[66,68,72] history of STD,[68] time as a CSW,[67,70,73] HIV infection,[72] and anal intercourse,[72] again supporting a link with sexual exposure.

Among STD clinic attendees, reported seroprevalence of HBV has ranged from 2% to 43%.[74–89] This wide range likely reflects different risk profiles and age of clinic attendees, and whether individuals originated from low-endemic versus intermediate-endemic or highly endemic HBV countries. Among studies of heterosexual STD clinic attendees that included controls, antibody to HBV core antigen was approximately 4 times higher than that observed among controls.[77–79] Sexual risk behaviors associated with HBV prevalence among these studies include number of sex partners,[74,77,86,88] past or current STD,[75,80,81,84,88,90,91] syphilis,[77,82] and years of sexual activity.[75,78,84]

Multiple countries have reported shifts in the epidemiology of HBV infection. Of acute hepatitis B cases admitted to hospital in Japan, transfusion-associated infection was seen only in the period from 1976 to 1990. From 1991 to 2002, sexual transmission accounted for 68% of cases, followed by infection at a medical facility or occupational exposure in 8%.[92] A case-control study of Taiwanese adults presenting with acute HBV found that heterosexual contact was the only reported risk in 83% of cases. Having a new sex partner appeared to be the most important factor associated with infection, and a direct relationship was observed between likelihood of HBV infection and number of sex partners.[93] For cases of acute hepatitis B reported in the United States in 2010 with risk factor information available, 28% reported 2 or more sex partners, 17% reported sex with another man, 8% indicated having sexual contact with a person with confirmed or suspected hepatitis B, 2% reported household contact with someone with confirmed or suspected of HBV infection, and 16% indicated injection drug use in the 6 weeks to 6 months before onset of symptoms. Less than 1% listed exposures via blood transfusion, dialysis, or occupational exposure.[94] Identifying and vaccinating adults at risk for hepatitis B plays a key role in reducing new adult hepatitis B infections in the United States.

MSM have long been recognized as a group with higher seroprevalence of HBV. Seroprevalence surveys of MSM in the 1980s found a prevalence of HBV infection of nearly 70%.[81,95,96] Among 2946 MSM living in the Netherlands, 4.8% were found to be HBsAg positive versus 0.22% among a large group of Dutch blood donors. Acquisition of HBV among 316 MSM tested in follow-up was 27.6% per year.[19] Among MSM followed in MACS (Multicenter AIDS Cohort Study) in Pittsburgh, HBV seroconversion was 19.8% over a 30-month follow-up period versus HIV-1 acquisition of 7.8%. Insertive anal intercourse was the major risk factor identified for HBV acquisition.[97] The Young Men's Survey,[98] a cross-sectional anonymous survey of 3432 MSM aged 15 to 22 years in US metropolitan areas conducted from 1994 to 1998, found past or current HBV infection, based on presence of antihepatitis core antibody (HBcAb) or HBsAg, in 11% of men sampled, ranging from 2% among 15-year-olds to 17% among 22-year-olds. Phase 2 of the Young Men's Survey[99] enrolled 2834 MSM aged 23 to 29 years from 1998 to 2000 and found seromarkers of HBV infection in 20.6% of participants, including 2.3% who had current or chronic infection. These data again supported a linear increase of HBV prevalence with age, with seroprevalence in phase 2 ranging from 13.7% in 23-year-olds to 31.1% in 29-year-olds. HBV infection was associated with a history of having an STD, having a greater number of lifetime partners, ever using injection drugs, and ever engaging in anal intercourse. Among HIV-negative MSM recruited from community and clinic settings for participation in the Canadian Omega Study in 1996 to 1997, 41% were found to have any marker of HBV (HBcAb, HBsAg, hepatitis B surface antibody [HBsAb]). Presence of HBV markers was associated with age, history of ulcerative STDs, injection drug use, having a partner with HIV, history of gonorrhea or chlamydia, number of partners, and receiving money for sex.[100] Similar to studies in heterosexual populations, STD clinic attendees, and CSW, risks for HBV in MSM have been associated with sexual behaviors and STDs. Identified risks include the duration of MSM activity,[14,86,101,102] past or present STDs,[81,99,100,102–106] syphilis,[13,95,104,106,107] HIV,[104,107] number of partners,[14,99–101,103,107,108] oral-anal sex,[101,102] and anal intercourse.[14,97,99,101,102]

Prevention of Hepatitis B

Currently available hepatitis B vaccines are highly effective at preventing HBV infection. Hepatitis B vaccine was first licensed in 1982, and recombinant vaccine was introduced in 1986. A 3-dose series generates a protective response in more than 90% of healthy vaccinees and provides long-lasting protection.[109–113] After completion of a vaccine series, an HBsAb level of 10 mIU/mL or greater is considered protective. In general, protection generated by a complete vaccine series is believed to last for at least 15 to 20 years in healthy individuals. Immunity in healthy adults and children seems to persist even although antibody levels may decline over time to low levels, even lower than detectable limits.[114–122]

In the United States, hepatitis B vaccine has been recommended for persons at high-risk of acquiring HBV since vaccine became available in 1982.[123] In 1991, the US Centers for Disease Control and Prevention (CDC) expanded recommendations to include universal immunization of all infants and specifically recommended vaccine for all MSM and for high-risk heterosexual men and women, defined as those who engage in commercial sex work, have been diagnosed with a recently acquired STD, or report 2 or more sex partners in the past 6 months.[124] Current recommendations for hepatitis B vaccination in US adults are based on known risks for HBV acquisition; specific health care evaluation, or treatment settings (in which a high proportion of clients have known risk factors for hepatitis B infection); and persons in whom hepatitis B infection would have significant health impact, including those with chronic liver disease or HIV infection, as detailed in **Box 1**.[125] Country-specific recommendations outside the United States vary, although the World Health Organization recommends universal HBV immunization of all infants starting at birth and supports additional target groups for catch-up vaccination appropriate to the epidemiologic setting and available resources.[54]

Two single-antigen vaccines (Engerix-B and Recombivax HB) and 1 combination antigen vaccine (TWINRIX, combined hepatitis A and B) are licensed for adults in the United States. All vaccines use HBsAg as the antigen. In the United States, recombinant DNA technology is used to generate HBsAg for all vaccines, and the vaccines do not contain thimerosal (or contain only trace amounts from the manufacturing process). The recommended schedules and dosing for hepatitis B vaccination are shown in **Box 2** and **Table 2**. Additional information on frequently asked questions regarding hepatitis B vaccine can be found at: http://www.cdc.gov/hepatitis/HBV/HBVfaq.htm (Hepatitis B FAQs for Health Professionals).

Despite the recognition that certain adult populations remain at risk for HBV infection through sexual transmission and the availability of a highly effective vaccine to prevent HBV infection, immunization rates among at-risk adults remain low.[52,87,98–100,106,126–134] In a recent national survey of physician practices for hepatitis B vaccination, only 31% of primary care physicians reported routinely assessing for and vaccinating adults who reported risk factors for hepatitis B infection.[126] Data from the US National Health Interview Survey from 2000 to 2009 were used to assess self-reported HBV vaccine coverage among 18-year-olds to 49-year-olds. In 2000, only 30% and 31% of high-risk men and women, respectively, reported having received at least 1 dose of hepatitis B vaccine despite more than 80% of high-risk adults reporting visits to a clinician during the past year.[129] By 2009, 50.5% of high-risk adults had received 1 or more doses of HBV vaccine, which constituted a 5% increase in vaccine coverage compared with 2004.[132] Although vaccine coverage increased, 50% of high-risk adults remained unvaccinated.

Among MSM aged 15 to 22 years surveyed in 1994 to 1998 in the Young Men's Health Study,[98] only 9% had serologic evidence of having received hepatitis B vaccine, despite

---

Box 1
Adults recommended to receive hepatitis B vaccine in the United States

Persons at risk for infection by sexual exposure

- Sex partners of HBsAg-positive persons
- Sexually active persons who are not in a long-term mutually monogamous relationship (eg, person with >1 sex partner during the previous 6 months)
- Persons seeking evaluation or treatment of a sexually transmitted disease
- MSM

Persons at risk for infection by percutaneous or mucosal exposure to blood

- Current or recent IDU
- Household contacts of HBsAg-positive persons
- Residents and staff of facilities for developmentally disabled persons
- Health care and public safety workers with reasonably anticipated risk for exposure to blood or blood-contaminated body fluids
- Persons with end-stage renal disease, including predialysis, hemodialysis, peritoneal dialysis, and home dialysis patients

Others

- International travelers to regions with high or intermediate levels (HBsAg prevalence >2%) of endemic HBV infection
- Persons with chronic liver disease
- Persons with HIV infection
- All other persons seeking protection from HBV infection

Data from Mast EE, Weinbaum CM, Fiore AE, et al. A comprehensive immunization strategy to eliminate transmission of hepatitis B virus infection in the United States, Recommendations of the Advisory Committee on Immunization Practices (ACIP) Part II: immunization of adults. MMWR Recomm Rep 2006;55(RR-16):1–25.

Box 2
Hepatitis B vaccine schedule (months) for adults (aged ≥20 years)[a]

0, 1, and 6

0, 1, and 4

0, 2, and 4

0, 1, 2, and 12[b]

[a] All schedules are applicable to single-antigen hepatitis B vaccines; TWINRIX (combined hepatitis A and hepatitis B vaccine) may be administered at 0, 1, and 6 months.
[b] A 4-dose schedule of Engerix-B is licensed for all age groups.
Data from Mast EE, Weinbaum CM, Fiore AE, et al. A comprehensive immunization strategy to eliminate transmission of hepatitis B virus infection in the United States, Recommendations of the Advisory Committee on Immunization Practices (ACIP) Part II: immunization of adults. MMWR Recomm Rep 2006;55(RR-16):1–25. Available at: ww.cdc.gov/mmwr/preview/mmwrhtml/rr5516a1.htm. Accessed April 3, 2013.

Table 2
Recommended doses of currently licensed formulations of hepatitis B vaccine, by age group and vaccine type

| | | Single-Antigen Vaccine | | | | Combination Vaccine | |
| | | Recombivax HB | | Engerix-B | | TWINRIX[a] | |
Age Group (y)		Dose (μg)[b]	Volume (mL)	Dose (μg)	Volume (mL)	Dose (μg)	Volume (mL)
Adolescents	11–15	10[c]	1.0	NA	NA	NA	NA
	11–19	5	0.5	10	0.5	NA	NA
Adults	≥20	10	1.0	20	1.0	10[a]	1.0
Hemodialysis or other immunocompromised persons	<20[d]	5	0.5	10	0.5	NA	NA
	≥20	40[e]	1.0	40[f]	2.0	NA	NA

Abbreviation: NA, not applicable.
  [a] Combined hepatitis A and hepatitis B vaccine is recommended for persons aged 18 years who are at increased risk for both hepatitis B and hepatitis A infections.
  [b] Recombinant HBsAg protein dose.
  [c] Adult formulation administered on a 2-dose schedule separated by at least 4 months is licensed for use in 11-year-olds to 15-year-olds.
  [d] Higher doses may be more immunogenic, but no specific recommendations have been made.
  [e] Dialysis formulation administered on a 3-dose schedule at 0, 1, and 6 months.
  [f] Two 1.0-mL doses administered at 1 site, on a 4-dose schedule at 0, 1, 2, and 6 months.
  Data from CDC FAQs for Health Professionals. Available at: http://www.cdc.gov/hepatitis/HBV/HBVfaq.htm. Accessed April 3, 2013.

more than 96% of those susceptible to hepatitis B having reported contact with the health care system, which included testing for HIV or receiving treatment of an STD. Seventy-seven percent of those surveyed were susceptible to HBV infection, and 11% had prevalent infection. Vaccine coverage among 23-year-olds to 29-year-olds surveyed in 1998 to 2000, was similarly low, with only 17% having evidence of vaccine-induced immunity. Surveys of MSM outside the United States have reported challenges with vaccine coverage in multiple settings, including MSM enrolled in a prospective cohort in Canada (48% reported ≥1 dose of vaccine),[100] in a cross-sectional study of MSM in the Netherlands (50% received ≥1 dose of vaccine),[135] and among a cross-sectional survey of MSM in Beijing (39% with seroevidence of immunity).[106] HBV vaccine coverage remains low even among HIV-infected persons attending urban HIV clinics in the United States[52] and among participants in the HIV Outpatient Study cohort.[131]

The low rate of HBV immunization in these instances represents missed opportunities to provide vaccination to adults at high risk of acquiring hepatitis B. When asked, most at-risk persons are willing to accept hepatitis B vaccination.[51,136–139] In addition to recommending and implementing routine hepatitis B vaccination for known at-risk populations, health care providers can identify persons in need of vaccination through an open, nonjudgmental discussion of sexual practices and risks for HBV acquisition. Person at risk should be counseled regarding their potential risk for HBV acquisition, the health impact of HBV infection, the availability of a highly effective vaccine, and other potential means to reduce risk (ie, consistent use of condoms and other effective barrier methods during vaginal, anal, and oral-anal sex; limiting or modifying high-risk sexual practices; limiting number of partners).

HEPATITIS C

Hepatitis C virus (HCV) is a common infection.[140] The CDC estimate that in the United States, 1.3% to 1.9% of the population has been infected with HCV, 2.7 million to 3.9 million people are living with chronic HCV infection, and approximately 12,000 deaths related to chronic HCV infection occur each year. Only a few of these infections are associated with an acute clinical illness.[94,141–143] HCV is transmitted primarily through percutaneous exposure, including injection drug use, receipt of blood or blood products, occupational percutaneous exposures, and potential nosocomial transmission in health care settings with inadequate infection control. Other less efficient routes of transmission include mother-to-child transmission and sexual transmission between partners. The contribution of sexual transmission to HCV acquisition has been debated and likely varies by the type of partnership and sexual practices between partners.

Sexual Transmission of HCV Among Heterosexual Partnerships

The presence of HCV in long-term partners of chronically HCV-infected persons has been studied in multiple settings, most frequently among cohorts of men with hemophilia or persons attending clinics for treatment of HCV. Seroprevalence of HCV among partners in these settings has ranged from 0% to 27%, with most studies showing seroprevalence in partners of less than 10%.[144–154] Higher HCV seroprevalence in partners has been more frequently reported from Southeast Asia and southern Europe than in northern Europe and the United States.[155] After adjusting for concordant genotypes in couples, seroprevalence estimates decline.[155]

Several prospective studies examined HCV transmission in long-term heterosexual partnerships.[151,156–161] Three cohorts reported no confirmed HCV transmission events between partners, including 1 study that had extended follow-up to 10 years.[151,157,158] The reported incidence of HCV infection was otherwise low, ranging from 2.3 to 12.0 per 1000 person-years.[156,160] Few studies included molecular analysis to confirm the presence of the same virus within infected partnerships.[145,156] Interpretation of these data may be confounded by factors such as the duration of relationship; the duration and intensity of sexual exposure; the relatively low-risk populations studied; and the potential for other shared risk factors, such as drug use, shared syringes, shared personal care items, resulting in blood exposure, and shared exposures in health care settings.

Heterosexual transmission of HCV may occur more efficiently in the presence of other biological and behavioral risks. Multiple studies have shown links between HIV infection and HCV prevalence.[162–166] Among HIV-infected women with no history of injection drug use participating in the Women's Interagency HIV Study,[165] sex with a male IDU was associated with prevalent HCV, and among all participants, being HIV infected was associated with a nearly 2-fold increased risk of being HCV coinfected. In a prospective cohort of non-IDUs, being HIV infected was associated with HCV prevalence.[164] Other identified potential risks for sexually acquired HCV include multiple sex partners,[163,166–168] high-risk sexual practices (ie, anonymous partners, sex in the setting of drug use, exchanging sex for money/drugs, sex with IDU),[169,170] presence or history of other STIs,[166,171–175] and exposure to blood via partner violence.[176]

Sexual Transmission of HCV Among MSM

Multiple reports have identified clusters of acute HCV infection among MSM, primarily among MSM who are coinfected with HIV.[177–181] Several other prospective cohorts and retrospective studies of HIV-infected persons or persons attending STD clinics have reported similar findings among HIV-infected MSM.[175,182–189] Although ongoing injection drug use remained the strongest risk factor for new HCV acquisition in several studies,[184,188,190] multiple case-control and cohort studies identified sexual contact as a potential source of transmission.[177,178,180,182,183,191,192] Two comprehensive reviews have recently been published on the topic of sexual transmission of hepatitis C.[193,194]

Among clinic-based samples of MSM, many have noted an increase in new HCV infections among attendees. Screening for HCV in these studies was not always universal, nor was follow-up completed in a prospective fashion; therefore, incidence estimates may be imprecise. However, they do contribute a useful perspective on the emergence of HCV in the community. In a retrospective study of HIV-infected MSM attending STD services in Antwerp,[186] annual incidence of HCV infection increased from 0.2% in 2001 to 1.5% in 2008 and 2.9% in 2009. A retrospective cohort of HIV-infected MSM attending sexual health services between 2002 and 2010 in Melbourne, Australia[190] calculated HCV incidence among non-IDU at 0.6/100 person-years. MSM participating in the Amsterdam Cohort Studies from 1984 to 2003 were retrospectively tested for HCV. Overall HCV incidence was 0.18 per 100 person-years in HIV-infected MSM versus zero seroconversions in HIV-negative MSM. HCV incidence among HIV-infected men increased from 0.08 per 100 person-years in 1984 to 1999 to 0.87 per 100 person-years in 2000 to 2003. MSM hospitalized with acute HCV after 2000 reported high rates of ulcerative STIs (59%) in the 6 months before HCV diagnosis and rough sexual techniques (55%), and all denied injection drug use.[182] Among HIV-infected MSM attending genitourinary medicine clinics in London and Brighton from 2002 to 2006,[195] overall estimated HCV incidence was 9.05 per 1000 patient-years, increasing from 6.86 per 1000 in 2002 to 11.58 per 1000 in 2006. This finding translated to an average annual increase in incidence of HCV of 20%. There was little evidence of transmission among MSM with negative or unknown HIV status. In contrast, a community-based sample of HIV-infected MSM in Sydney saw no incident HCV infections from 2001 to 2007 among those tested. Baseline HCV seropositivity was 9.4% and was strongly associated with a history of IDU.[196]

Several prospective studies have noted an increase in HCV infection among HIV-infected MSM. Among MSM enrolled in a large HIV seroconverters cohort, the Concerted Action on SeroConversion to AIDS and Death in Europe (CASCADE) Collaboration,[183] incidence of HCV in 1990 was low at 0.9 to 2.2 per 100 person-years, increasing to 5.5 to 8.1 per 1000 person-years in 1995. Incidence increased substantially after 2002, increasing to 16.8 to 30.0 per 1000 person-years in 2005 and 23.4 to 51.1 per 1000 person-years in 2007. Within the prospective Swiss HIV Cohort,[187] incidence rates of HCV among MSM increased from 0.23 per 100 person-years in 1998 to 4.09 per 100 person-years in 2011, with 51 of 101 total cases occurring in the previous 3 years. In contrast, HCV among IDUs over the same period decreased from 13.89 to 2.24 per 100 years, with only 3 incident cases in the previous 3 years. HCV acquisition among heterosexuals remained low at less than 0.5 per 100 person-years. Among MSM, inconsistent condom use and past syphilis infection predicted HCV seroconversion. When examining HCV incidence among subsets of MSM in this cohort, incidence among non-IDU MSM reporting unsafe sexual practices was 0.7 per 100 person-years, higher than that seen among non-IDU MSM not reporting unsafe sex (0.2 per 100 person-years) and non-IDU heterosexuals (0.18 per 100 person-years).[184] Among HIV-infected men and women enrolled in the French PRIMO Cohort,[185] overall HCV incidence was 3.5 and 7.8 per 100 person-years among men and women respectively, with a trend toward rising incidence from 2003 to 2006. The only identified risk factor for HCV acquisition among men was unsafe sex. Recent data from an observational cohort of HIV-infected non-IDUs in Taiwan[175] reported increasing HCV incidence in MSM enrollees, with rates increasing from 0 in 1994 to 2000 to 3.49 per 1000 person-years in 2001 to 2005 to 12.32 per 1000 person-years in 2006 to 2010. After adjustment for age and HIV transmission route, recent syphilis infection remained an independent factor associated with HCV seroconversion. HCV incidence was evaluated in a long-term cohort of HIV-infected men participating in a US-based clinical trial (AIDS Clinical Trial Group Longitudinal Linked Randomized Trials cohort) contributing more than 7000 person-years of follow-up. Overall incidence was 0.51 per 100 person-years, with incidence higher among IDU (2.67 per 100 person-years) versus non-IDU (0.40 per 100 person-years). However, 75% of seroconverters reported no IDU. Seroconversion was associated with HIV RNA levels of greater than 400 copies/mL. Individual-level behavioral risk data were not available.[197] In a national sample of HIV-infected MSM attending HIV care in France,[198] HCV incidence was estimated at 4.8 per 1000 in 2006 and 3.6 per 1000 in 2007. Most men with HCV reported higher-risk sexual practices in the 6 months before HCV diagnosis, including multiple partners, partners sought online or at sex venues, unprotected anal sex, bleeding during sex, fisting, and recreational drug use.

Among HIV-infected MSM who have been previously diagnosed and successfully treated for acute HCV infection, sporadic cases of recurrent HCV infection, documented by a switch in infecting genotype or clade, have been documented. The only reported risk in the 2 cases of reinfection was unprotected anal intercourse with multiple HIV-infected male partners.[199] Among 56 men followed after treatment of HCV, 5 relapsed and 11 became reinfected, with a median time to reinfection of 8.4 months. There was a cumulative 33% reinfection rate after 2 years. Report of non-injecting recreational drug use was identified as a risk for reinfection. No difference in reported sexual behaviors was found.[200]

HCV prevalence and incidence among HIV-negative MSM without a history of injection drug use seem to still be low,[182,189,195,201,202] although there have been reports of presumed sexually acquired HCV infection among these men.[196,203] A prospective study of MSM in Canada, the Omega Cohort,[202] found baseline HCV prevalence at entry of 2.9%, which was strongly linked to injection drug use. Overall HCV incidence in the cohort was 0.038 per 100 person-years, with the single seroconversion occurring in an active IDU. Within the Amsterdam Cohort Studies of MSM followed from 1984 to 2003,[182] no HCV seroconversions were observed in HIV-negative MSM, despite a corresponding increase in incidence among HIV-positive MSM. Among HIV-negative MSM recruited in a community-based setting in Sydney in 2001 to 2007,[16] baseline HCV prevalence was 1.1%, with an incidence of 0.11 per 100 person-years. Four of the 5 seroconverters reported sexual contact with HIV-positive men and 2 had an incident ulcerative STI. MSM attending a public STD clinic in the United Kingdom from 2000 to 2006,[189] where the clinic policy was to perform regular HCV screening in all MSM, were found to have an HCV incidence of 1.5 per 1000 person-years in HIV-negative MSM versus 11.8 per 100 person-years in HIV-positive MSM. New HCV diagnoses increased annually among both HIV-infected men and among men whose HIV status was negative or unknown. A recent systematic review of HCV infection in HIV-positive and HIV-negative MSM provided pooled incidence estimates of HCV infection in HIV-negative MSM of 1.48/1000 person-years (95% confidence interval 0.75–2.21) versus 6.08/1000 person-years (95% confidence interval 5.18–6.99) in HIV-positive MSM.[204]

Factors associated with potential sexual transmission of HCV among MSM identified across multiple studies are:

- Coinfection with HIV[205–207]
- Unprotected anal intercourse, especially as the receptive partner[177,178,185,191,198,206,208–210]

- Inconsistent condom use[187]
- Use of recreational drugs/drug use during sex[177,192,200,207,210]
- Current or previous STIs, especially ulcerative STIs including lymphogranuloma venereum proctitis, syphilis, and herpes simplex[175,178,180,182,185,187,196,206,209]
- Multiple or anonymous/casual sex partners[178,191,198,199,210]
- Group sex[191,192]
- Sexual practices that result in bleeding or damage to mucosa; fisting; and use of shared sex toys[178,180,191,192,198,206–210]

The use of molecular epidemiology has defined HCV transmission clusters within MSM networks, further detailing sexual transmission in this group.[179,182,191,198,211–213] In a study of HIV-infected MSM with acute HCV identified in urban HIV clinics in the United Kingdom,[191] case HCV sequences were compared with unrelated reference sequences. Seven genetically distinct HCV variants were found to be cocirculating in the HIV-positive MSM cases. Four of the 7 clusters had origins in the mid-1990s, with most (64%) of all lineage divergences occurring since 1995, implying increased transmission from this time point. Phylogenetic analysis of HCV isolates from HIV-infected MSM enrolled in a French study of acute HCV infection (HEPAIG)[198] reported 4 distinct clusters, which were distinct from sequences obtained from French IDU or other French patients. HIV-infected MSM with acute HCV subtype 4d identified in Germany were found to comprise 2 MSM-specific clusters distinct from circulating IDU and non-MSM clusters. All except 1 of the German MSM belonged to a large MSM-specific HCV cluster containing MSM from 4 different European countries.[211] An international phylogenetic analysis of 226 HCV isolates from HIV-infected MSM with recent HCV infection in the United Kingdom, France, Germany, Australia, and the Netherlands[179] reported a large international network of HCV transmission among HIV-positive MSM, with 84% of MSM having an HCV strain that was most similar to HCV present in another MSM participant in the study. A large proportion (74%) of European MSM was infected with an HCV strain cocirculating in multiple European countries. Molecular clock analysis indicated that most (85%) of the transmissions had occurred since 1996. ATAHC (Australian Trial in Acute Hepatitis C)[213] included persons infected via injection drug use (73%) and via sexual transmission (18%). Among 112 individuals whose HCV isolates were sequenced, 23 (20%) were infected with a strain of HCV identical to that of another subject, most of which (78%) were HIV infected. Fifty-one percent of HIV-infected individuals had a virus that was homologous with another individual, compared with only 8% of HIV-uninfected individuals. Clusters contained individuals with both injection drug use-related and sex-related acquisition risks and MSM, suggesting that both injection and sexual route of transmission were active within the same social networks.

Most current HCV transmission in MSM seems to be among HIV-infected persons and remains an ongoing problem. Although even HIV-uninfected MSM may be at increased risk for HCV acquisition in the setting of higher-risk sexual practices or partnerships with HIV/HCV-positive partners. Several biological and behavioral factors have been linked to HCV transmission among MSM, including HIV coinfection; participation in sexual practices that result in mucosal damage or result in exposure to blood; presence of STIs, particularly ulcerative STIs; multiple/casual sex partners; and unprotected anal intercourse. HIV-infected persons should be tested for HCV at entry to care[214,215] and then assessed at regular intervals for risk factors related to acquisition of new HCV infection. Although injection drug use remains the strongest predictor for new HCV infection among HIV-infected persons, there is increasing evidence of sexual transmission of HCV among MSM engaging in higher-risk sexual practices, prompting some organizations to recommend regular HCV screening for HIV-infected MSM.[216] Discussing sexual and drug-use practices can help identify persons at risk for HCV acquisition and prompt rescreening for HCV infection. The possibility of HCV infection in patients presenting with symptoms suggestive of acute hepatitis or with newly increased liver function tests should be performed as part of a comprehensive evaluation.

Prevention of Hepatitis C

There is no vaccine for the prevention of hepatitis C. Although the risk for sexually transmitting hepatitis C is probably low if blood is not involved, the consistent use of condoms for sexual activity can reduce the risk of STI in general, including HIV and hepatitis B. People with chronic hepatitis C should discuss the risk of hepatitis C transmission, which is low but not absent, with their sex partners. Using latex condoms and minimizing sexual exposure to blood should reduce the risk of sexual transmission. Although injection drug use remains the strongest predictor for new HCV infection, there is increasing evidence for sexual transmission of HCV among HIV-infected MSM engaging in higher-risk sexual practices. An open conversation regarding sexual and drug-use practices and methods to potentially reduce the risk of sexually acquired HCV (limiting of number of sex partners, use of barrier methods, avoiding or limiting identified high-risk sexual practices) should be discussed. No intervention studies have addressed methods to reduce HCV sexual transmission.

SUMMARY

Epidemiologic and molecular data support the role of sexual contact in transmission of hepatitis A, B, and C. Although there is little evidence to suggest that sexual contact plays a significant role in transmission of hepatitis A among heterosexual partners, outbreaks and regional transmission of hepatitis A do occur among MSM. Hepatitis A vaccine is the most effective means of prevention among at-risk adults. Hepatitis B (HBV) is efficiently transmitted through sexual contact between men and women and between MSM. Identification and vaccination of adults at risk for HBV acquisition through sexual contact is a key strategy to reduce new HBV infections among at-risk adults; however, effective implementation of hepatitis B immunization in at-risk adults remains a challenge. Transmission of HCV through heterosexual contact seems to be inefficient, with previous studies showing transmission among long-term monogamous heterosexual partners occurring in less than 1% of couples per year. Heterosexual transmission of HCV may occur more efficiently in the presence of other biological and behavioral risks, including HIV coinfection, higher-risk sexual practices, and in the presence of other STIs. Hepatitis C has emerged as an STI among MSM, primarily among MSM who are HIV infected. Several factors have been linked to HCV transmission among MSM, including HIV coinfection; participation in sexual practices that result in mucosal damage or result in exposure to blood; presence of STIs, particularly ulcerative STIs; multiple/casual sex partners; and unprotected anal intercourse. Provider awareness of the potential for sexual transmission of viral hepatitis, an open discussion with patients regarding sexual partners and practices that may place them at risk, and routinely offering available preventive vaccine to at-risk adults has the potential to reduce morbidity and mortality from these common infections.

REFERENCES

1. Tassopoulos NC, Papaevangelou GJ, Ticehurst JR, et al. Fecal excretion of Greek strains of hepatitis A virus in patients with hepatitis A and in experimentally infected chimpanzees. J Infect Dis 1986;154(2):231–7.

2. Robertson BH, Averhoff F, Cromeans TL, et al. Genetic relatedness of hepatitis A virus isolates during a community-wide outbreak. J Med Virol 2000;62(2): 144–50.
3. Staes CJ, Schlenker TL, Risk I, et al. Sources of infection among persons with acute hepatitis A and no identified risk factors during a sustained community-wide outbreak. Pediatrics 2000;106(4):E54.
4. Victor JC, Surdina TY, Suleimenova SZ, et al. Person-to-person transmission of hepatitis A virus in an urban area of intermediate endemicity: implications for vaccination strategies. Am J Epidemiol 2006;163(3):204–10.
5. Venczel LV, Desai MM, Vertz PD, et al. The role of child care in a community-wide outbreak of hepatitis A. Pediatrics 2001;108(5):E78.
6. Smith PF, Grabau JC, Werzberger A, et al. The role of young children in a community-wide outbreak of hepatitis A. Epidemiol Infect 1997;118(3):243–52.
7. Ross JD, Ghanem M, Tariq A, et al. Seroprevalence of hepatitis A immunity in male genitourinary medicine clinic attenders: a case control study of heterosexual and homosexual men. Sex Transm Infect 2002;78(3):174–9.
8. Corona R, Stroffolini T, Giglio A, et al. Lack of evidence for increased risk of hepatitis A infection in homosexual men. Epidemiol Infect 1999;123(1):89–93.
9. Nandwani R, Caswell S, Boag F, et al. Hepatitis A seroprevalence in homosexual and heterosexual men. Genitourin Med 1994;70(5):325–8.
10. McFarlane ES, Embil JA, Manuel FR, et al. Antibodies to hepatitis A antigen in relation to the number of lifetime sexual partners in patients attending an STD clinic. Br J Vener Dis 1981;57(1):58–61.
11. McFarlane ES, Embil JA, Manuel FR, et al. Prevalence of antibodies to hepatitis A antigen in patients attending a clinic for treatment of sexually transmitted diseases. Sex Transm Dis 1980;7(2):87–9.
12. Ballesteros J, Dal-Re R, Gonzalez A, et al. Are homosexual males a risk group for hepatitis A infection in intermediate endemicity areas? Epidemiol Infect 1996; 117(1):145–8.
13. Kryger P, Pedersen NS, Mathiesen L, et al. Increased risk of infection with hepatitis A and B viruses in men with a history of syphilis: relation to sexual contacts. J Infect Dis 1982;145(1):23–6.
14. Coester CH, Avonts D, Colaert J, et al. Syphilis, hepatitis A, hepatitis B, and cytomegalovirus infection in homosexual men in Antwerp. Br J Vener Dis 1984;60(1):48–51.
15. Corey L, Holmes KK. Sexual transmission of hepatitis A in homosexual men: incidence and mechanism. N Engl J Med 1980;302(8):435–8.
16. Jin F, Prestage GP, Zablotska I, et al. High rates of sexually transmitted infections in HIV positive homosexual men: data from two community based cohorts. Sex Transm Infect 2007;83(5):397–9.
17. Katz MH, Hsu L, Wong E, et al. Seroprevalence of and risk factors for hepatitis A infection among young homosexual and bisexual men. J Infect Dis 1997;175(5): 1225–9.
18. Villano SA, Nelson KE, Vlahov D, et al. Hepatitis A among homosexual men and injection drug users: more evidence for vaccination. Clin Infect Dis 1997;25(3): 726–8.
19. Coutinho RA, Albrecht-van Lent P, Lelie N, et al. Prevalence and incidence of hepatitis A among male homosexuals. Br Med J (Clin Res Ed) 1983; 287(6407):1743–5.
20. Kosatsky T, Middaugh JP. Linked outbreaks of hepatitis A in homosexual men and in food service patrons and employees. West J Med 1986;144(3):307–10.

21. Henning KJ, Bell E, Braun J, et al. A community-wide outbreak of hepatitis A: risk factors for infection among homosexual and bisexual men. Am J Med 1995;99(2):132–6.

22. Reintjes R, Bosman A, de Zwart O, et al. Outbreak of hepatitis A in Rotterdam associated with visits to 'darkrooms' in gay bars. Commun Dis Public Health 1999;2(1):43–6.

23. Bell A, Ncube F, Hansell A, et al. An outbreak of hepatitis A among young men associated with having sex in public venues. Commun Dis Public Health 2001; 4(3):163–70.

24. Mazick A, Howitz M, Rex S, et al. Hepatitis A outbreak among MSM linked to casual sex and gay saunas in Copenhagen, Denmark. Euro Surveill 2005; 10(5):111–4.

25. Christenson B, Brostrom C, Bottiger M, et al. An epidemic outbreak of hepatitis A among homosexual men in Stockholm. Hepatitis A, a special hazard for the male homosexual subpopulation in Sweden. Am J Epidemiol 1982;116(4): 599–607.

26. Cotter SM, Sansom S, Long T, et al. Outbreak of hepatitis A among men who have sex with men: implications for hepatitis A vaccination strategies. J Infect Dis 2003;187(8):1235–40.

27. Leentvaar-Kuijpers A, Kool JL, Veugelers PJ, et al. An outbreak of hepatitis A among homosexual men in Amsterdam, 1991-1993. Int J Epidemiol 1995; 24(1):218–22.

28. Stewart T, Crofts N. An outbreak of hepatitis A among homosexual men in Melbourne. Med J Aust 1993;158(8):519–21.

29. Stokes ML, Ferson MJ, Young LC. Outbreak of hepatitis A among homosexual men in Sydney. Am J Public Health 1997;87(12):2039–41.

30. Sundkvist T, Aitken C, Duckworth G, et al. Outbreak of acute hepatitis A among homosexual men in East London. Scand J Infect Dis 1997;29(3):211–2.

31. Walsh B, Sundkvist T, Maguire H, et al. Rise in hepatitis A among gay men in the Thames regions 1995 and 1996. Genitourin Med 1996;72(6):449–50.

32. Takechi A, Hatakeyama S, Kashiyama T, et al. Outbreak of hepatitis A virus infection among men who have sex with men. Kansenshogaku Zasshi 2000; 74(9):716–9 [in Japanese].

33. Centers for Disease Control (CDC). Hepatitis A among homosexual men–United States, Canada, and Australia. MMWR Morb Mortal Wkly Rep 1992;41:155, 61–4.

34. Centers for Disease Control (CDC). Hepatitis A vaccination of men who have sex with men–Atlanta, Georgia, 1996-1997. MMWR Morb Mortal Wkly Rep 1998; 47(34):708–11.

35. Roy E, Haley N, Leclerc P, et al. Seroprevalence and risk factors for hepatitis A among Montreal street youth. Can J Public Health 2002;93(1):52–3.

36. van Steenbergen JE, Tjon G, van den Hoek A, et al. Two years' prospective collection of molecular and epidemiological data shows limited spread of hepatitis A virus outside risk groups in Amsterdam, 2000-2002. J Infect Dis 2004; 189(3):471–82.

37. Tjon G, Xiridou M, Coutinho R, et al. Different transmission patterns of hepatitis A virus for two main risk groups as evidenced by molecular cluster analysis. J Med Virol 2007;79(5):488–94.

38. Stene-Johansen K, Tjon G, Schreier E, et al. Molecular epidemiological studies show that hepatitis A virus is endemic among active homosexual men in Europe. J Med Virol 2007;79(4):356–65.

39. Fiore AE, Wasley A, Bell BP. Prevention of hepatitis A through active or passive immunization: recommendations of the Advisory Committee on Immunization Practices (ACIP). MMWR Recomm Rep 2006;55(RR-7):1–23.
40. McMahon BJ, Williams J, Bulkow L, et al. Immunogenicity of an inactivated hepatitis A vaccine in Alaska Native children and Native and non-Native adults. J Infect Dis 1995;171(3):676–9.
41. Clemens R, Safary A, Hepburn A, et al. Clinical experience with an inactivated hepatitis A vaccine. J Infect Dis 1995;171(Suppl 1):S44–9.
42. Van Herck K, Van Damme P, Lievens M, et al. Hepatitis A vaccine: indirect evidence of immune memory 12 years after the primary course. J Med Virol 2004;72(2):194–6.
43. Hess G, Clemens R, Bienzle U, et al. Immunogenicity and safety of an inactivated hepatitis A vaccine in anti-HIV positive and negative homosexual men. J Med Virol 1995;46(1):40–2.
44. Neilsen GA, Bodsworth NJ, Watts N. Response to hepatitis A vaccination in human immunodeficiency virus-infected and -uninfected homosexual men. J Infect Dis 1997;176(4):1064–7.
45. Kemper CA, Haubrich R, Frank I, et al. Safety and immunogenicity of hepatitis A vaccine in human immunodeficiency virus-infected patients: a double-blind, randomized, placebo-controlled trial. J Infect Dis 2003;187(8):1327–31.
46. Wallace MR, Brandt CJ, Earhart KC, et al. Safety and immunogenicity of an inactivated hepatitis A vaccine among HIV-infected subjects. Clin Infect Dis 2004; 39(8):1207–13.
47. Rimland D, Guest JL. Response to hepatitis A vaccine in HIV patients in the HAART era. AIDS 2005;19(15):1702–4.
48. Prevention of hepatitis A through active or passive immunization: recommendations of the Advisory Committee on Immunization Practices (ACIP). MMWR Recomm Rep 1996;45(RR-15):1–30.
49. Prevention of hepatitis A through active or passive immunization: recommendations of the Advisory Committee on Immunization Practices (ACIP). MMWR Recomm Rep 1999;48(RR-12):1–37.
50. National Advisory Committee on Immunization, Public Health Agency of Canada. Canadian Immunization Guide, Evergreen Edition. 2012. Available at: http://www.phac-aspc.gc.ca/publicat/cig-gci/index-eng.php. Accessed March 16, 2013.
51. Sansom S, Rudy E, Strine T, et al. Hepatitis A and B vaccination in a sexually transmitted disease clinic for men who have sex with men. Sex Transm Dis 2003;30(9):685–8.
52. Hoover KW, Butler M, Workowski KA, et al. Low rates of hepatitis screening and vaccination of HIV-infected MSM in HIV clinics. Sex Transm Dis 2012;39(5):349–53.
53. Gay and Lesbian Medical Association. Study shows: hepatitis vaccination rates on the rise among gay and bisexual men but fewer than 50% are fully protected. 2004. Available at: http://www.glma.org/index.cfm?fuseaction=Feature.showFeature&CategoryID=4&FeatureID=41. Accessed March 16, 2013.
54. World Health Organization. Hepatitis B vaccines: WHO Position Paper. Weekly Epidemiological Record 2009;40(84):405–20.
55. Goldstein ST, Zhou F, Hadler SC, et al. A mathematical model to estimate global hepatitis B disease burden and vaccination impact. Int J Epidemiol 2005;34(6):1329–39.
56. Ayoola EA, Odelola HA, Ladipo OA. Hepatitis B surface antigen in menstrual blood and semen. Int J Gynaecol Obstet 1980;18(3):185–7.

57. Berry WR, Gottesfeld RL, Alter HJ, et al. Transmission of hepatitis B virus by artificial insemination. JAMA 1987;257(8):1079–81.
58. Karayiannis P, Novick DM, Lok AS, et al. Hepatitis B virus DNA in saliva, urine, and seminal fluid of carriers of hepatitis B e antigen. Br Med J (Clin Res Ed) 1985;290(6485):1853–5.
59. Inaba N, Ohkawa R, Matsuura A, et al. Sexual transmission of hepatitis B surface antigen. Infection of husbands by HBsAg carrier-state wives. Br J Vener Dis 1979;55(5):366–8.
60. Men BY, Xu HW, Wang XL. Hepatitis B surface antigen (HBsAg) in feces of convalescent hepatitis B patients. Chin Med J (Engl) 1989;102(8):596–9.
61. Reiner NE, Judson FN, Bond WW, et al. Asymptomatic rectal mucosal lesions and hepatitis B surface antigen at sites of sexual contact in homosexual men with persistent hepatitis B virus infection. Ann Intern Med 1982;96(2):170–3.
62. Scott RM, Snitbhan R, Bancroft WH, et al. Experimental transmission of hepatitis B virus by semen and saliva. J Infect Dis 1980;142(1):67–71.
63. Alter HJ, Purcell RH, Gerin JL, et al. Transmission of hepatitis B to chimpanzees by hepatitis B surface antigen-positive saliva and semen. Infect Immun 1977; 16(3):928–33.
64. Koff RS, Slavin MM, Connelly JD, et al. Contagiousness of acute hepatitis B. Secondary attack rates in household contacts. Gastroenterology 1977;72(2): 297–300.
65. Redeker AG, Mosley JW, Gocke DJ, et al. Hepatitis B immune globulin as a prophylactic measure for spouses exposed to acute type B hepatitis. N Engl J Med 1975;293(21):1055–9.
66. Bratos MA, Eiros JM, Orduna A, et al. Influence of syphilis in hepatitis B transmission in a cohort of female prostitutes. Sex Transm Dis 1993;20(5):257–61.
67. Goh CL, Rajan VS, Chan SH, et al. Hepatitis B infection in prostitutes. Int J Epidemiol 1986;15(1):112–5.
68. Hyams KC, Escamilla J, Lozada Romero R, et al. Hepatitis B infection in a non-drug abusing prostitute population in Mexico. Scand J Infect Dis 1990;22(5): 527–31.
69. Hyams KC, Phillips IA, Tejada A, et al. Three-year incidence study of retroviral and viral hepatitis transmission in a Peruvian prostitute population. J Acquir Immune Defic Syndr 1993;6(12):1353–7.
70. Hyams KC, Phillips IA, Tejada A, et al. Hepatitis B in a highly active prostitute population: evidence for a low risk of chronic antigenemia. J Infect Dis 1990; 162(2):295–8.
71. Lurie P, Fernandes ME, Hughes V, et al. Socioeconomic status and risk of HIV-1, syphilis and hepatitis B infection among sex workers in Sao Paulo State, Brazil. Instituto Adolfo Lutz Study Group. AIDS 1995;9(Suppl 1):S31–7.
72. Rosenblum L, Darrow W, Witte J, et al. Sexual practices in the transmission of hepatitis B virus and prevalence of hepatitis delta virus infection in female prostitutes in the United States. JAMA 1992;267(18):2477–81.
73. Van Doornum GJ, Van Haastrecht HJ, Hooykaas C, et al. Hepatitis B virus infection in a group of heterosexuals with multiple partners in Amsterdam, The Netherlands: implications for vaccination? J Med Virol 1994;43(1):20–7.
74. Alter MJ, Ahtone J, Weisfuse I, et al. Hepatitis B virus transmission between heterosexuals. JAMA 1986;256(10):1307–10.
75. Baddour LM, Bucak VA, Somes G, et al. Risk factors for hepatitis B virus infection in black female attendees of a sexually transmitted disease clinic. Sex Transm Dis 1988;15(3):174–6.

76. Christopher PJ, Crewe EB, Mailer PT, et al. Hepatitis B infection among STD clinic patients in Sydney. Aust N Z J Med 1984;14(4):491–4.

77. Corona R, Caprilli F, Giglio A, et al. Risk factors for hepatitis B virus infection among heterosexuals attending a sexually transmitted diseases clinic in Italy: role of genital ulcerative diseases. J Med Virol 1996;48(3):262–6.

78. el-Dalil AA, Jayaweera DT, Walzman M, et al. Hepatitis B markers in heterosexual patients attending two genitourinary medicine clinics in the West Midlands. Genitourin Med 1997;73(2):127–30.

79. Gilson RJ, de Ruiter A, Waite J, et al. Hepatitis B virus infection in patients attending a genitourinary medicine clinic: risk factors and vaccine coverage. Sex Transm Infect 1998;74(2):110–5.

80. Kvinesdal BB, Worm AM, Gottschau A. Risk factors for hepatitis B virus infection in heterosexuals attending a venereal disease clinic in Copenhagen. Scand J Infect Dis 1993;25(2):171–5.

81. Mele A, Franco E, Caprilli F, et al. Hepatitis B and delta virus infection among heterosexuals, homosexuals and bisexual men. Eur J Epidemiol 1988;4(4): 488–91.

82. Oliveira LH, Silva IR, Xavier BL, et al. Hepatitis B infection among patients attending a sexually transmitted diseases clinic in Rio de Janeiro, Brazil. Mem Inst Oswaldo Cruz 2001;96(5):635–40.

83. Risbud A, Mehendale S, Basu S, et al. Prevalence and incidence of hepatitis B virus infection in STD clinic attendees in Pune, India. Sex Transm Infect 2002; 78(3):169–73.

84. Romanowski B, Campbell P. Sero-epidemiologic study to determine the prevalence and risk of hepatitis B in a Canadian heterosexual sexually transmitted disease population. Can J Public Health 1994;85(3):205–7.

85. Smith HM, Alexander GJ, Webb G, et al. Hepatitis B and delta virus infection among "at risk" populations in south east London. J Epidemiol Community Health 1992;46(2):144–7.

86. Szmuness W, Much I, Prince AM, et al. On the role of sexual behavior in the spread of hepatitis B infection. Ann Intern Med 1975;83(4):489–95.

87. Trepka MJ, Weisbord JS, Zhang G, et al. Hepatitis B virus infection risk factors and immunity among sexually transmitted disease clinic clients. Sex Transm Dis 2003;30(12):914–8.

88. van Duynhoven YT, van de Laar MJ, Schop WA, et al. Prevalence and risk factors for hepatitis B virus infections among visitors to an STD clinic. Genitourin Med 1997;73(6):488–92.

89. Barrett CL, Austin H, Louv WC, et al. Risk factors for hepatitis B virus infection among women attending a clinic for sexually transmitted diseases. Sex Transm Dis 1992;19(1):14–8.

90. Hart G. Factors associated with hepatitis B infection. Int J STD AIDS 1993;4(2): 102–6.

91. Hentzer B, Skinhoj P, Hoybye G, et al. Viral hepatitis in a venereal clinic population. Relation to certain risk factors. Scand J Infect Dis 1980;12(4): 245–9.

92. Arima S, Michitaka K, Horiike N, et al. Change of acute hepatitis B transmission routes in Japan. J Gastroenterol 2003;38(8):772–5.

93. Hou MC, Wu JC, Kuo BI, et al. Heterosexual transmission as the most common route of acute hepatitis B virus infection among adults in Taiwan–the importance of extending vaccination to susceptible adults. J Infect Dis 1993; 167(4):938–41.

94. Centers for Disease Control and Prevention, Division of Viral Hepatitis. Viral Hepatitis Surveillance–United States, 2010, August 20, 2012. Available at: http://www.cdc.gov/hepatitis/Statistics/2010Surveillance/index.htm.

95. Bleeker A, Coutinho RA, Bakker-Kok J, et al. Prevalence of syphilis and hepatitis B among homosexual men in two saunas in Amsterdam. Br J Vener Dis 1981; 57(3):196–9.

96. Hess G, Bienzle U, Slusarczyk J, et al. Hepatitis B virus and delta infection in male homosexuals. Liver 1986;6(1):13–6.

97. Kingsley LA, Rinaldo CR Jr, Lyter DW, et al. Sexual transmission efficiency of hepatitis B virus and human immunodeficiency virus among homosexual men. JAMA 1990;264(2):230–4.

98. MacKellar DA, Valleroy LA, Secura GM, et al. Two decades after vaccine license: hepatitis B immunization and infection among young men who have sex with men. Am J Public Health 2001;91(6):965–71.

99. Weinbaum CM, Lyerla R, Mackellar DA, et al. The Young Men's Survey phase II: hepatitis B immunization and infection among young men who have sex with men. Am J Public Health 2008;98(5):839–45.

100. Remis RS, Dufour A, Alary M, et al. Association of hepatitis B virus infection with other sexually transmitted infections in homosexual men. Omega Study Group. Am J Public Health 2000;90(10):1570–4.

101. Schreeder MT, Thompson SE, Hadler SC, et al. Hepatitis B in homosexual men: prevalence of infection and factors related to transmission. J Infect Dis 1982; 146(1):7–15.

102. Osella AR, Massa MA, Joekes S, et al. Hepatitis B and C virus sexual transmission among homosexual men. Am J Gastroenterol 1998;93(1):49–52.

103. Jin F, Prestage GP, Pell CM, et al. Hepatitis A and B infection and vaccination in a cohort of homosexual men in Sydney. Sex Health 2004;1(4):227–37.

104. Lama JR, Agurto HS, Guanira JV, et al. Hepatitis B infection and association with other sexually transmitted infections among men who have sex with men in Peru. Am J Trop Med Hyg 2010;83(1):194–200.

105. Seage GR 3rd, Mayer KH, Lenderking WR, et al. HIV and hepatitis B infection and risk behavior in young gay and bisexual men. Public Health Rep 1997; 112(2):158–67.

106. Wang C, Wang Y, Huang X, et al. Prevalence and factors associated with hepatitis B immunization and infection among men who have sex with men in Beijing, China. PLoS One 2012;7(10):e48219.

107. Stroffolini T, Corona R, Giglio A, et al. Risk factors for hepatitis B virus infection among homosexual men attending a sexually transmitted diseases clinic in Italy. New Microbiol 1997;20(4):333–8.

108. Lim KS, Wong VT, Fulford KW, et al. Role of sexual and non-sexual practices in the transmission of hepatitis B. Br J Vener Dis 1977;53(3):190–2.

109. Andre FE. Summary of safety and efficacy data on a yeast-derived hepatitis B vaccine. Am J Med 1989;87(3A):14S–20S.

110. Zajac BA, West DJ, McAleer WJ, et al. Overview of clinical studies with hepatitis B vaccine made by recombinant DNA. J Infect 1986;13(Suppl A):39–45.

111. Szmuness W, Stevens CE, Zang EA, et al. A controlled clinical trial of the efficacy of the hepatitis B vaccine (Heptavax B): a final report. Hepatology 1981; 1(5):377–85.

112. Francis DP, Hadler SC, Thompson SE, et al. The prevention of hepatitis B with vaccine. Report of the centers for disease control multi-center efficacy trial among homosexual men. Ann Intern Med 1982;97(3):362–6.

113. Krugman S, Holley HP Jr, Davidson M, et al. Immunogenic effect of inactivated hepatitis B vaccine: comparison of 20 microgram and 40 microgram doses. J Med Virol 1981;8(2):119–21.
114. Fitzsimons D, Francois G, Hall A, et al. Long-term efficacy of hepatitis B vaccine, booster policy, and impact of hepatitis B virus mutants. Vaccine 2005;23(32):4158–66.
115. Bauer T, Jilg W. Hepatitis B surface antigen-specific T and B cell memory in individuals who had lost protective antibodies after hepatitis B vaccination. Vaccine 2006;24(5):572–7.
116. Jack AD, Hall AJ, Maine N, et al. What level of hepatitis B antibody is protective? J Infect Dis 1999;179(2):489–92.
117. Williams IT, Goldstein ST, Tufa J, et al. Long term antibody response to hepatitis B vaccination beginning at birth and to subsequent booster vaccination. Pediatr Infect Dis J 2003;22(2):157–63.
118. Lin YC, Chang MH, Ni YH, et al. Long-term immunogenicity and efficacy of universal hepatitis B virus vaccination in Taiwan. J Infect Dis 2003;187(1):134–8.
119. Zanetti AR, Mariano A, Romano L, et al. Long-term immunogenicity of hepatitis B vaccination and policy for booster: an Italian multicentre study. Lancet 2005;366(9494):1379–84.
120. Boxall EH, A Sira J, El-Shuhkri N, et al. Long-term persistence of immunity to hepatitis B after vaccination during infancy in a country where endemicity is low. J Infect Dis 2004;190(7):1264–9.
121. Wang RX, Boland GJ, van Hattum J, et al. Long-term persistence of T cell memory to HBsAg after hepatitis B vaccination. World J Gastroenterol 2004;10(2):260–3.
122. Yuen MF, Lim WL, Chan AO, et al. 18-year follow-up study of a prospective randomized trial of hepatitis B vaccinations without booster doses in children. Clin Gastroenterol Hepatol 2004;2(10):941–5.
123. Centers for Disease Control (CDC). Recommendation of the Immunization Practices Advisory Committee (ACIP). Inactivated hepatitis B virus vaccine. MMWR Morb Mortal Wkly Rep 1982;31(24):317–22, 27–8.
124. Hepatitis B virus: a comprehensive strategy for eliminating transmission in the United States through universal childhood vaccination. Recommendations of the Immunization Practices Advisory Committee (ACIP). MMWR Recomm Rep 1991;40(RR-13):1–25.
125. Mast EE, Weinbaum CM, Fiore AE, et al. A comprehensive immunization strategy to eliminate transmission of hepatitis B virus infection in the United States: recommendations of the Advisory Committee on Immunization Practices (ACIP) Part II: immunization of adults. MMWR Recomm Rep 2006;55(RR-16):1–33 [quiz: CE1–4].
126. Daley MF, Hennessey KA, Weinbaum CM, et al. Physician practices regarding adult hepatitis B vaccination: a national survey. Am J Prev Med 2009;36(6):491–6.
127. Centers for Disease Control (CDC). Undervaccination for hepatitis B among young men who have sex with men–San Francisco and Berkeley, California, 1992-1993. MMWR Morb Mortal Wkly Rep 1996;45(10):215–7.
128. Centers for Disease Control (CDC). Hepatitis B vaccination among high-risk adolescents and adults–San Diego, California, 1998-2001. MMWR Morb Mortal Wkly Rep 2002;51(28):618–21.
129. Jain N, Yusuf H, Wortley PM, et al. Factors associated with receiving hepatitis B vaccination among high-risk adults in the United States: an analysis of the National Health Interview Survey, 2000. Fam Med 2004;36(7):480–6.

130. Dufour A, Remis RS, Alary M, et al. Factors associated with hepatitis B vaccination among men having sexual relations with men in Montreal, Quebec, Canada. Omega Study Group. Sex Transm Dis 1999;26(6):317–24.
131. Spradling PR, Richardson JT, Buchacz K, et al. Prevalence of chronic hepatitis B virus infection among patients in the HIV Outpatient Study, 1996-2007. J Viral Hepat 2010;17(12):879–86.
132. Lu PJ, Byrd KK, Murphy TV, et al. Hepatitis B vaccination coverage among high-risk adults 18-49 years, U.S., 2009. Vaccine 2011;29(40):7049–57.
133. Harris JL, Jones TS, Buffington J. Hepatitis B vaccination in six STD clinics in the United States committed to integrating viral hepatitis prevention services. Public Health Rep 2007;122(Suppl 2):42–7.
134. Gilbert LK, Bulger J, Scanlon K, et al. Integrating hepatitis B prevention into sexually transmitted disease services: U.S. sexually transmitted disease program and clinic trends–1997 and 2001. Sex Transm Dis 2005;32(6):346–50.
135. Baars JE, Boon BJ, Garretsen HF, et al. The reach of a hepatitis B vaccination programme among men who have sex with men. Eur J Public Health 2011; 21(3):333–7.
136. Bhatti N, Gilson RJ, Beecham M, et al. Failure to deliver hepatitis B vaccine: confessions from a genitourinary medicine clinic. BMJ 1991;303(6794):97–101.
137. McCusker J, Hill EM, Mayer KH. Awareness and use of hepatitis B vaccine among homosexual male clients of a Boston community health center. Public Health Rep 1990;105(1):59–64.
138. Samoff E, Dunn A, VanDevanter N, et al. Predictors of acceptance of hepatitis B vaccination in an urban sexually transmitted diseases clinic. Sex Transm Dis 2004;31(7):415–20.
139. van Steenbergen JE. Results of an enhanced-outreach programme of hepatitis B vaccination in the Netherlands (1998-2000) among men who have sex with men, hard drug users, sex workers and heterosexual persons with multiple partners. J Hepatol 2002;37(4):507–13.
140. Shepard CW, Finelli L, Alter MJ. Global epidemiology of hepatitis C virus infection. Lancet Infect Dis 2005;5(9):558–67.
141. Armstrong GL, Wasley A, Simard EP, et al. The prevalence of hepatitis C virus infection in the United States, 1999 through 2002. Ann Intern Med 2006; 144(10):705–14.
142. Daniels D, Grytdal S, Wasley A. Surveillance for acute viral hepatitis–United States, 2007. MMWR Surveill Summ 2009;58(3):1–27.
143. Mitchell AE, Colvin HM, Palmer Beasley R. Institute of Medicine recommendations for the prevention and control of hepatitis B and C. Hepatology 2010; 51(3):729–33.
144. Akahane Y, Aikawa T, Sugai Y, et al. Transmission of HCV between spouses. Lancet 1992;339(8800):1059–60.
145. Chayama K, Kobayashi M, Tsubota A, et al. Molecular analysis of intraspousal transmission of hepatitis C virus. J Hepatol 1995;22(4):431–9.
146. Kao JH, Hwang YT, Chen PJ, et al. Transmission of hepatitis C virus between spouses: the important role of exposure duration. Am J Gastroenterol 1996; 91(10):2087–90.
147. Neumayr G, Propst A, Schwaighofer H, et al. Lack of evidence for the heterosexual transmission of hepatitis C. QJM 1999;92(9):505–8.
148. Stroffolini T, Lorenzoni U, Menniti-Ippolito F, et al. Hepatitis C virus infection in spouses: sexual transmission or common exposure to the same risk factors? Am J Gastroenterol 2001;96(11):3138–41.

149. Sun CA, Chen HC, Lu CF, et al. Transmission of hepatitis C virus in Taiwan: prevalence and risk factors based on a nationwide survey. J Med Virol 1999;59(3): 290–6.
150. Hisada M, O'Brien TR, Rosenberg PS, et al. Virus load and risk of heterosexual transmission of human immunodeficiency virus and hepatitis C virus by men with hemophilia. The Multicenter Hemophilia Cohort Study. J Infect Dis 2000; 181(4):1475–8.
151. Tahan V, Karaca C, Yildirim B, et al. Sexual transmission of HCV between spouses. Am J Gastroenterol 2005;100(4):821–4.
152. Scotto G, Savastano AM, Fazio V, et al. Sexual transmission of hepatitis C virus infection. Eur J Epidemiol 1996;12(3):241–4.
153. Bresters D, Mauser-Bunschoten EP, Reesink HW, et al. Sexual transmission of hepatitis C virus. Lancet 1993;342(8865):210–1.
154. Brettler DB, Mannucci PM, Gringeri A, et al. The low risk of hepatitis C virus transmission among sexual partners of hepatitis C-infected hemophilic males: an international, multicenter study. Blood 1992;80(2):540–3.
155. Terrault NA. Sexual activity as a risk factor for hepatitis C. Hepatology 2002; 36(5 Suppl 1):S99–105.
156. Kao JH, Liu CJ, Chen PJ, et al. Low incidence of hepatitis C virus transmission between spouses: a prospective study. J Gastroenterol Hepatol 2000;15(4):391–5.
157. Marincovich B, Castilla J, del Romero J, et al. Absence of hepatitis C virus transmission in a prospective cohort of heterosexual serodiscordant couples. Sex Transm Infect 2003;79(2):160–2.
158. Vandelli C, Renzo F, Romano L, et al. Lack of evidence of sexual transmission of hepatitis C among monogamous couples: results of a 10-year prospective follow-up study. Am J Gastroenterol 2004;99(5):855–9.
159. Riestra S, Fernandez E, Rodriguez M, et al. Hepatitis C virus infection in heterosexual partners of HCV carriers. J Hepatol 1995;22(4):509–10.
160. Piazza M, Sagliocca L, Tosone G, et al. Sexual transmission of the hepatitis C virus and efficacy of prophylaxis with intramuscular immune serum globulin. A randomized controlled trial. Arch Intern Med 1997;157(14):1537–44.
161. Wyld R, Robertson JR, Brettle RP, et al. Absence of hepatitis C virus transmission but frequent transmission of HIV-1 from sexual contact with doubly-infected individuals. J Infect 1997;35(2):163–6.
162. Giuliani M, Caprilli F, Gentili G, et al. Incidence and determinants of hepatitis C virus infection among individuals at risk of sexually transmitted diseases attending a human immunodeficiency virus type 1 testing program. Sex Transm Dis 1997;24(9):533–7.
163. Daikos GL, Lai S, Fischl MA. Hepatitis C virus infection in a sexually active inner city population. The potential for heterosexual transmission. Infection 1994; 22(2):72–6.
164. Van Den Berg CH, Van De Laar TJ, Kok A, et al. Never injected, but hepatitis C virus-infected: a study among self-declared never-injecting drug users from the Amsterdam Cohort Studies. J Viral Hepat 2009;16(8):568–77.
165. Frederick T, Burian P, Terrault N, et al. Factors associated with prevalent hepatitis C infection among HIV-infected women with no reported history of injection drug use: the Women's Interagency HIV Study (WIHS). AIDS Patient Care STDS 2009;23(11):915–23.
166. Thomas DL, Zenilman JM, Alter HJ, et al. Sexual transmission of hepatitis C virus among patients attending sexually transmitted diseases clinics in Baltimore–an analysis of 309 sex partnerships. J Infect Dis 1995;171(4):768–75.

167. Salleras L, Bruguera M, Vidal J, et al. Importance of sexual transmission of hepatitis C virus in seropositive pregnant women: a case-control study. J Med Virol 1997;52(2):164–7.
168. Mele A, Tosti ME, Marzolini A, et al. Prevention of hepatitis C in Italy: lessons from surveillance of type-specific acute viral hepatitis. SEIEVA collaborating Group. J Viral Hepat 2000;7(1):30–5.
169. Feldman JG, Minkoff H, Landesman S, et al. Heterosexual transmission of hepatitis C, hepatitis B, and HIV-1 in a sample of inner city women. Sex Transm Dis 2000;27(6):338–42.
170. Wang CC, Krantz E, Klarquist J, et al. Acute hepatitis C in a contemporary US cohort: modes of acquisition and factors influencing viral clearance. J Infect Dis 2007;196(10):1474–82.
171. Page-Shafer KA, Cahoon-Young B, Klausner JD, et al. Hepatitis C virus infection in young, low-income women: the role of sexually transmitted infection as a potential cofactor for HCV infection. Am J Public Health 2002;92(4):670–6.
172. Hershow RC, Kalish LA, Sha B, et al. Hepatitis C virus infection in Chicago women with or at risk for HIV infection: evidence for sexual transmission. Sex Transm Dis 1998;25(10):527–32.
173. Shev S, Hermodsson S, Lindholm A, et al. Risk factor exposure among hepatitis C virus RNA positive Swedish blood donors–the role of parenteral and sexual transmission. Scand J Infect Dis 1995;27(2):99–104.
174. Marx MA, Murugavel KG, Tarwater PM, et al. Association of hepatitis C virus infection with sexual exposure in southern India. Clin Infect Dis 2003;37(4): 514–20.
175. Sun HY, Chang SY, Yang ZY, et al. Recent hepatitis C virus infections in HIV-infected patients in Taiwan: incidence and risk factors. J Clin Microbiol 2012;50(3):781–7.
176. Russell M, Chen MJ, Nochajski TH, et al. Risky sexual behavior, bleeding caused by intimate partner violence, and hepatitis C virus infection in patients of a sexually transmitted disease clinic. Am J Public Health 2009;99(Suppl 1): S173–9.
177. Centers for Disease Control (CDC). Sexual transmission of hepatitis C virus among HIV-infected men who have sex with men–New York City, 2005-2010. MMWR Morb Mortal Wkly Rep 2011;60(28):945–50.
178. Gambotti L, Batisse D, Colin-de-Verdiere N, et al. Acute hepatitis C infection in HIV positive men who have sex with men in Paris, France, 2001-2004. Euro Surveill 2005;10(5):115–7.
179. van de Laar T, Pybus O, Bruisten S, et al. Evidence of a large, international network of HCV transmission in HIV-positive men who have sex with men. Gastroenterology 2009;136(5):1609–17.
180. Gotz HM, van Doornum G, Niesters HG, et al. A cluster of acute hepatitis C virus infection among men who have sex with men–results from contact tracing and public health implications. AIDS 2005;19(9):969–74.
181. van de Laar TJ, Matthews GV, Prins M, et al. Acute hepatitis C in HIV-infected men who have sex with men: an emerging sexually transmitted infection. AIDS 2010;24(12):1799–812.
182. van de Laar TJ, van der Bij AK, Prins M, et al. Increase in HCV incidence among men who have sex with men in Amsterdam most likely caused by sexual transmission. J Infect Dis 2007;196(2):230–8.
183. van der Helm JJ, Prins M, del Amo J, et al. The hepatitis C epidemic among HIV-positive MSM: incidence estimates from 1990 to 2007. AIDS 2011;25(8): 1083–91.

184. Rauch A, Rickenbach M, Weber R, et al. Unsafe sex and increased incidence of Hepatitis C virus infection among HIV-infected men who have sex with men: the Swiss HIV Cohort Study. Clin Infect Dis 2005;41(3):395–402.
185. Ghosn J, Deveau C, Goujard C, et al. Increase in hepatitis C virus incidence in HIV-1-infected patients followed up since primary infection. Sex Transm Infect 2006;82(6):458–60.
186. Bottieau E, Apers L, Van Esbroeck M, et al. Hepatitis C virus infection in HIV-infected men who have sex with men: sustained rising incidence in Antwerp, Belgium, 2001-2009. Euro Surveill 2010;15(39):19673.
187. Wandeler G, Gsponer T, Bregenzer A, et al. Hepatitis C virus infections in the Swiss HIV Cohort Study: a rapidly evolving epidemic. Clin Infect Dis 2012;55(10):1408–16.
188. Taylor LE, Holubar M, Wu K, et al. Incident hepatitis C virus infection among US HIV-infected men enrolled in clinical trials. Clin Infect Dis 2011;52(6):812–8.
189. Richardson D, Fisher M, Sabin CA. Sexual transmission of hepatitis C in MSM may not be confined to those with HIV infection. J Infect Dis 2008;197(8):1213–4 [author reply: 4–5].
190. Gamage DG, Read TR, Bradshaw CS, et al. Incidence of hepatitis-C among HIV infected men who have sex with men (MSM) attending a sexual health service: a cohort study. BMC Infect Dis 2011;11:39.
191. Danta M, Brown D, Bhagani S, et al. Recent epidemic of acute hepatitis C virus in HIV-positive men who have sex with men linked to high-risk sexual behaviours. AIDS 2007;21(8):983–91.
192. Schmidt AJ, Rockstroh JK, Vogel M, et al. Trouble with bleeding: risk factors for acute hepatitis C among HIV-positive gay men from Germany–a case-control study. PLoS One 2011;6(3):e17781.
193. Tohme RA, Holmberg SD. Is sexual contact a major mode of hepatitis C virus transmission? Hepatology 2010;52(4):1497–505.
194. Danta M, Dusheiko GM. Acute HCV in HIV-positive individuals–a review. Curr Pharm Des 2008;14(17):1690–7.
195. Giraudon I, Ruf M, Maguire H, et al. Increase in diagnosed newly acquired hepatitis C in HIV-positive men who have sex with men across London and Brighton, 2002–2006: is this an outbreak? Sex Transm Infect 2008;84(2):111–5.
196. Jin F, Prestage GP, Matthews G, et al. Prevalence, incidence and risk factors for hepatitis C in homosexual men: data from two cohorts of HIV-negative and HIV-positive men in Sydney, Australia. Sex Transm Infect 2010;86(1):25–8.
197. Taylor L, Holubar M, Wu K, et al. Incident hepatitis C virus infection among US HIV-infected men enrolled in clinical trials. Clin Infect Dis 2011;52(6):812–8.
198. Larsen C, Chaix ML, Le Strat Y, et al. Gaining greater insight into HCV emergence in HIV-infected men who have sex with men: the HEPAIG Study. PLoS One 2011;6(12):e29322.
199. Cotte L, Chevallier Queyron P, Schlienger I, et al. Sexually transmitted HCV infection and reinfection in HIV-infected homosexual men. Gastroenterol Clin Biol 2009;33(10–11):977–80.
200. Lambers FA, Prins M, Thomas X, et al. Alarming incidence of hepatitis C virus (HCV) reinfection after treatment of sexually acquired acute HCV infection in HIV-infected men having sex with men in Amsterdam. AIDS 2011;25(17):F21–7.
201. Buffington J, Murray PJ, Schlanger K, et al. Low prevalence of hepatitis C virus antibody in men who have sex with men who do not inject drugs. Public Health Rep 2007;122(Suppl 2):63–7.

202. Alary M, Joly JR, Vincelette J, et al. Lack of evidence of sexual transmission of hepatitis C virus in a prospective cohort study of men who have sex with men. Am J Public Health 2005;95(3):502–5.
203. van de Laar TJ, Paxton WA, Zorgdrager F, et al. Sexual transmission of hepatitis C virus in human immunodeficiency virus-negative men who have sex with men: a series of case reports. Sex Transm Dis 2011;38(2):102–4.
204. Yaphe S, Bozinoff N, Kyle R, et al. Incidence of acute hepatitis C virus infection among men who have sex with men with and without HIV infection: a systematic review. Sex Transm Infect 2012;88(7):558–64.
205. Bodsworth NJ, Cunningham P, Kaldor J, et al. Hepatitis C virus infection in a large cohort of homosexually active men: independent associations with HIV-1 infection and injecting drug use but not sexual behaviour. Genitourin Med 1996;72(2):118–22.
206. Buchbinder SP, Katz MH, Hessol NA, et al. Hepatitis C virus infection in sexually active homosexual men. J Infect 1994;29(3):263–9.
207. Urbanus AT, van de Laar TJ, Stolte IG, et al. Hepatitis C virus infections among HIV-infected men who have sex with men: an expanding epidemic. AIDS 2009; 23(12):F1–7.
208. Cohen DE, Russell CJ, Golub SA, et al. Prevalence of hepatitis C virus infection among men who have sex with men at a Boston community health center and its association with markers of high-risk behavior. AIDS Patient Care STDs 2006; 20(8):557–64.
209. Ndimbie OK, Kingsley LA, Nedjar S, et al. Hepatitis C virus infection in a male homosexual cohort: risk factor analysis. Genitourin Med 1996;72(3):213–6.
210. Turner JM, Rider AT, Imrie J, et al. Behavioural predictors of subsequent hepatitis C diagnosis in a UK clinic sample of HIV positive men who have sex with men. Sex Transm Infect 2006;82(4):298–300.
211. Vogel M, van de Laar T, Kupfer B, et al. Phylogenetic analysis of acute hepatitis C virus genotype 4 infections among human immunodeficiency virus-positive men who have sex with men in Germany. Liver Int 2010;30(8):1169–72.
212. Serpaggi J, Chaix ML, Batisse D, et al. Sexually transmitted acute infection with a clustered genotype 4 hepatitis C virus in HIV-1-infected men and inefficacy of early antiviral therapy. AIDS 2006;20(2):233–40.
213. Matthews GV, Pham ST, Hellard M, et al. Patterns and characteristics of hepatitis C transmission clusters among HIV-positive and HIV-negative individuals in the Australian trial in acute hepatitis C. Clin Infect Dis 2011;52(6):803–11.
214. Aberg JA, Kaplan JE, Libman H, et al. Primary care guidelines for the management of persons infected with human immunodeficiency virus: 2009 update by the HIV Medicine Association of the Infectious Diseases Society of America. Clin Infect Dis 2009;49(5):651–81.
215. Kaplan JE, Benson C, Holmes KH, et al. Guidelines for prevention and treatment of opportunistic infections in HIV-infected adults and adolescents: recommendations from CDC, the National Institutes of Health, and the HIV Medicine Association of the Infectious Diseases Society of America. MMWR Recomm Rep 2009; 58(RR-4):1–207 [quiz: CE1–4].
216. European AIDS Treatment Network (NEAT) Acute Hepatitis C Infection Consensus Panel. Acute hepatitis C in HIV-infected individuals: recommendations from the European AIDS Treatment Network (NEAT) consensus conference. AIDS 2011; 25(4):399–409.

Index

Note: Page numbers of article titles are in **boldface** type.

A

Abscess(es)
  tubo-ovarian
    PID and, 801–802
Antimicrobial resistance
  in *Neisseria gonorrhoeae,* **723–737**. *See also Neisseria gonorrhoeae,* antimicrobial
    resistance in
Antimicrobial therapy
  for PID
    alternative regimens, 799–800
    CDC recommendations for, 798–799

B

Breastfeeding
  trichomoniasis during, 760

C

CDC. *See* Centers for Disease Control and Prevention (CDC)
Centers for Disease Control and Prevention (CDC)
  PID diagnostic criteria of
    sensitivity and specificity of, 796–797
  PID management recommendations of
    antimicrobial therapy–related, 798–799
Cephalosporin(s)
  contemporary resistance to, 725–726
  treatment failures with, 726–728
Cerebrospinal fluid (CSF) analysis
  in syphilis diagnosis, 715
Cervicitis
  genital chlamydial infections and
    in women, 740
Children
  trichomoniasis in, 761
Chlamydia trachomatis
  genital infections due to, 739
  PID due to, 794
Chlamydial infections
  genital, **739–753**. *See also specific types and* Genital chlamydial infections
Congenital syphilis
  clinical features of, 713
  diagnosis of, 715–716

Infect Dis Clin N Am 27 (2013) 837–843
http://dx.doi.org/10.1016/S0891-5520(13)00092-5
0891-5520/13/$ – see front matter © 2013 Elsevier Inc. All rights reserved.

id.theclinics.com

Congenital (*continued*)
     pregnancy and, 718
CSF analysis. *See* Cerebrospinal fluid (CSF) analysis

   E

Epididymitis
     genital chlamydial infections and
          in men, 741–742
Ethnicity
     as factor in genital chlamydial infections, 745

   G

Genital chlamydial infections, **739–753**
     causes of, 739
     clinical manifestations of
          in men, 741–743
               epididymitis, 741–742
               LGV, 743
               proctitis/proctocolitiis, 742
               prostatitis, 742
          in women, 740–741
               cervicitis, 740
               PID, 740–741
               urethritis, 740, 741
     diagnosis of, 743–744
     epidemiology of, 744–748
     follow-up care, 750
     introduction, 739
     race/ethnicity in, 745
     screening for, 744
     in sexual minority populations, 745–746
     treatment of, 748–750
     in young women, 745
Gonorrhea
     control of
          antimicrobial surveillance in, 724
          in era of evolving antimicrobial resistance, **723–737**. *See also Neisseria gonorrhoeae*
          introduction, 723–724
     diagnosis of, 728–730
     epidemiology of, 724
     prevalence of, 723–724
     screening for, 728–729
     treatment of, 730–733
          future options in, 731–732
          guidelines in, 730–731
          partner treatment in, 732
          rescreening in, 732
          test-of-cure in, 732
          vaccine in, 732–733
Gummatous syphilis, 713

H

HAV. *See* Hepatitis A virus (HAV)
HBV. *See* Hepatitis B virus (HBV)
HCV. *See* Hepatitis C virus (HCV)
Hepatitis
    viral. *See* Viral hepatitis
Hepatitis A virus (HAV)
    prevention of, 813–815
    sexual transmission of, 812–815
Hepatitis B virus (HBV)
    prevention of, 817–819
    sexual transmission of, 815–819
Hepatitis C virus (HCV)
    prevention of, 824
    sexual transmission of, 820–824
        among heterosexual partnerships, 820
        among MSM, 820–824
HIV infection
    Mycoplasma genitalium and, 783
    PID in women with, 802
    trichomoniasis and, 760
HPV. *See* Human papillomavirus (HPV)
Human papillomavirus (HPV), **765–778**
    background of, 765–766
    clinical features of, 768
    clinical management of, 770–771
    control of, 771–775
    diagnosis of, 768–770
    epidemiology of, 766–767
    magnitude of burden of, 766
    natural history of, 766–767
    prevention of, 771–775
    screening for, 768–770
    transmission of, 766–767
Human papillomavirus (HPV)–associated diseases, **765–778**. *See also* Human
    papillomavirus (HPV)
    natural history of, 767–768

I

Intrauterine devices (IUDs)
    PID in women using, 802
IUDs. *See* Intrauterine devices (IUDs)

L

LGV
    epidemiology of, 747–748
    genital chlamydial infections and
        in men, 743

M

Men who have sex with men (MSM)
   genital chlamydial infections in, 746
   HCV in
      sexual transmission of, 820–824
MSM. *See* Men who have sex with men (MSM)
Mycoplasma genitalium, **779–792**
   bacterium in, 780
   epidemiology of, 780–783
   future challenges related to, 784–785
   HIV and, 783
   introduction, 779–780
   treatment of, 783–784

N

NAAT
   in genital chlamydial infections diagnosis, 743–744
Neisseria gonorrhoeae. See also Gonorrhea
   antimicrobial resistance in
      evolution of, 725–728
      introduction, 723–724
      molecular mechanisms of, 728
   control of
      antimicrobial resistance in, **723–737**
   PID due to, 794

P

Pelvic inflammatory disease (PID), **793–809**
   causes of, 794
   CDC diagnostic criteria for
      sensitivity and specificity of, 796–797
   clinical evaluation of, 795–796
   described, 793
   differential diagnosis of, 795–796
   epidemiology of, 793–794
   genital chlamydial infections and
      in women, 740–741
   in HIV–infected women, 802
   imaging studies of, 797–798
   IUD use and, 802
   laboratory testing for, 797
   management of
      antimicrobial therapy in
         alternative regimens, 799–800
         CDC recommendations for, 798–799
      empiric coverage for anaerobic bacteria in, 800–801
      inpatient *vs.* outpatient, 798
   pathogenesis of, 794–795

in postmenopausal women, 802
    prevention of, 803
    sequelae associated with, 802–803
    in special populations, 802
    TOA and, 801–802
PID. *See* Pelvic inflammatory disease (PID)
Postmenopausal women
    PID in, 802
Pregnancy
    congenital syphilis and, 713
    trichomoniasis during, 760
Proctitis/proctocolitiis
    genital chlamydial infections and
        in men, 742
Prostatitis
    genital chlamydial infections and
        in men, 742

R

Race
    as factor in genital chlamydial infections, 745

S

Sexual minority(ies)
    genital chlamydial infections in, 745–746
Sexually transmitted diseases (STDs). *See specific types*
Syphilis
    cardiovascular, 713
    causes of, 705–706
    clinical features of, 708–713
        early syphilis, 708–711
            latent, 709–711
            primary, 708
            secondary, 708–709
        late syphilis, 711–713
            cardiovascular complications of, 713
            neurologic complications of, 711–712
            tertiary, 711
    congenital, 713
        diagnosis of, 715–716
        pregnancy and, 718
    diagnosis of, 713–716
        congenital syphilis, 715–716
        CSF analysis in, 715
        primary syphilis, 714
        secondary syphilis, 714–715
        tertiary syphilis, 715
    epidemiology of, 706–707
    follow-up care, 716–718

Syphilis (*continued*)
    gummatous, 713
    historical perspective of, 707
    incidence of, 706
    in modern era, **705–722**
    pathogenesis of, 705–706
    sex partners with
        management of, 718–719
    treatment of, 716

T

Test-of-cure
    in gonorrhea management, 732
TOA. *See* Tubo-ovarian abscess (TOA)
Treponema pallidum
    syphilis due to, 705
Trichomoniasis, **755–764**
    adverse outcomes of, 759–760
    during breastfeeding, 760
    in children, 761
    clinical management of, 758–759
    controversies related to, 761
    described, 755
    diagnosis of, 757–758
    epidemiology of, 755–756
    HIV and, 760
    introduction, 755
    pathophysiology of, 756–757
    in pregnancy, 760
    prevention of, 761
    special considerations, 760–761
Tubo-ovarian abscess (TOA)
    PID and, 801–802

U

Urethritis
    genital chlamydial infections and
        in men, 741
        in women, 740

V

Vaccine(s)
    for gonorrhea, 732–733
Viral hepatitis
    sexual transmission of, **811–836**
        HAV, 812–815
        HBV, 815–819
        HCV, 820–824

introduction, 811–812
  research related to, 812

W

Women who have sex with women (WSW)
  genital chlamydial infections in, 745–746

United States Postal Service

Statement of Ownership, Management, and Circulation
(All Periodicals Publications Except Requester Publications)

1. Publication Title	2. Publication Number		3. Filing Date
Infectious Disease Clinics of North America	0 0 1 - 5 5 6		9/14/13

4. Issue Frequency	5. Number of Issues Published Annually	6. Annual Subscription Price
Mar, Jun, Sep, Dec	4	$282.00

7. Complete Mailing Address of Known Office of Publication (Not printer) (Street, city, county, state, and ZIP+4®)

Elsevier Inc.
360 Park Avenue South
New York, NY 10010-1710

Contact Person
Stephen R. Bushing
Telephone (Include area code)
215-239-3688

8. Complete Mailing Address of Headquarters or General Business Office of Publisher (Not printer)

Elsevier Inc., 360 Park Avenue South, New York, NY 10010-1710

9. Full Names and Complete Mailing Addresses of Publisher, Editor, and Managing Editor (Do not leave blank)

Publisher (Name and complete mailing address)

Linda Belfus, Elsevier, Inc., 1600 John F. Kennedy Blvd. Suite 1800, Philadelphia, PA 19103-2899

Editor (Name and complete mailing address)

Stephanie Donley, Elsevier, Inc., 1600 John F. Kennedy Blvd. Suite 1800, Philadelphia, PA 19103-2899

Managing Editor (Name and complete mailing address)

Adrianne Brigido, Elsevier, Inc., 1600 John F. Kennedy Blvd. Suite 1800, Philadelphia, PA 19103-2899

10. Owner (Do not leave blank. If the publication is owned by a corporation, give the name and address of the corporation immediately followed by the names and addresses of all stockholders owning or holding 1 percent or more of the total amount of stock. If not owned by a corporation, give the names and addresses of the individual owners. If owned by a partnership or other unincorporated firm, give its name and address as well as those of each individual owner. If the publication is published by a nonprofit organization, give its name and address.)

Full Name	Complete Mailing Address
Wholly owned subsidiary of	1600 John F. Kennedy Blvd, Ste. 1800
Reed/Elsevier, US holdings	Philadelphia, PA 19103-2899

11. Known Bondholders, Mortgagees, and Other Security Holders Owning or Holding 1 Percent or More of Total Amount of Bonds, Mortgages, or Other Securities. If none, check box ☐ None

Full Name	Complete Mailing Address
N/A	

12. Tax Status (For completion by nonprofit organizations authorized to mail at nonprofit rates) (Check one)
The purpose, function, and nonprofit status of this organization and the exempt status for federal income tax purposes:
☐ Has Not Changed During Preceding 12 Months
☐ Has Changed During Preceding 12 Months (Publisher must submit explanation of change with this statement)

PS Form 3526, September 2007 (Page 1 of 3 (Instructions Page 3)) PSN 7530-01-000-9931 PRIVACY NOTICE: See our Privacy policy in www.usps.com

---

13. Publication Title	14. Issue Date for Circulation Data Below
Infectious Disease Clinics of North America	June 2013

15. Extent and Nature of Circulation

			Average No. Copies Each Issue During Preceding 12 Months	No. Copies of Single Issue Published Nearest to Filing Date
a. Total Number of Copies (Net press run)			802	727
b. Paid Circulation (By Mail and Outside the Mail)	(1)	Mailed Outside-County Paid Subscriptions Stated on PS Form 3541. (Include paid distribution above nominal rate, advertiser's proof copies, and exchange copies)	451	429
	(2)	Mailed In-County Paid Subscriptions Stated on PS Form 3541 (Include paid distribution above nominal rate, advertiser's proof copies, and exchange copies)		
	(3)	Paid Distribution Outside the Mails Including Sales Through Dealers and Carriers, Street Vendors, Counter Sales, and Other Paid Distribution Outside USPS®	117	118
	(4)	Paid Distribution by Other Classes Mailed Through the USPS (e.g. First-Class Mail®)		
c. Total Paid Distribution (Sum of 15b (1), (2), (3), and (4))			568	547
d. Free or Nominal Rate Distribution (By Mail and Outside the Mail)	(1)	Free or Nominal Rate Outside-County Copies Included on PS Form 3541	51	30
	(2)	Free or Nominal Rate In-County Copies Included on PS Form 3541		
	(3)	Free or Nominal Rate Copies Mailed at Other Classes Through the USPS (e.g. First-Class Mail)		
	(4)	Free or Nominal Rate Distribution Outside the Mail (Carriers or other means)		
e. Total Free or Nominal Rate Distribution (Sum of 15d (1), (2), (3) and (4))			51	30
f. Total Distribution (Sum of 15c and 15e)			619	577
g. Copies not Distributed (See instructions to publishers #4 (page #3))			183	150
h. Total (Sum of 15f and g)			802	727
i. Percent Paid (15c divided by 15f times 100)			91.76%	94.80%

16. Publication of Statement of Ownership
☐ If the publication is a general publication, publication of this statement is required. Will be printed in the December 2013 issue of this publication. ☐ Publication not required.

17. Signature and Title of Editor, Publisher, Business Manager, or Owner

Stephen R. Bushing
Stephen R. Bushing -Inventory Distribution Coordinator

Date: September 14, 2013

I certify that all information furnished on this form is true and complete. I understand that anyone who furnishes false or misleading information on this form or who omits material or information requested on the form may be subject to criminal sanctions (including fines and imprisonment) and/or civil sanctions (including civil penalties).

PS Form 3526, September 2007 (Page 2 of 3)